The Family Fitness Fun Book

The Family Fitness Fun Book

Healthy Living for the Whole Family

Rose R. Kennedy

healthyliving**books**

New York

Hatherleigh Press
5-22 46th Avenue, Suite 200
Long Island City, NY 11101
1-800-528-2550
www.hatherleighpress.com

Hatherleigh Press books are available for bulk purchase, special promotions and premiums. For more information on reselling and special purchase opportunities, please call us at 1-800-528-2550, and ask for the Special Sales Manager.

Library of Congress Cataloging-in-Publication Data

Kennedy, Rose.
  Family fitness fun book : healthy living for the whole family / Rose Kennedy.
       p. cm.
  ISBN 1-57826-145-7
  1. Family recreation. 2. Physical fitness. 3. Games. I. Title.
  GV182.8.K45 2005
  790.1'91—dc22
                                        2005001930

Interior design and layout by Deborah Miller
Cover design by Phil Mondestin and Deborah Miller

10 9 8 7 6 5 4 3 2 1
Printed in the United States

DEDICATION

To every child who ever played on Matoaka Court in Williamsburg, Virginia, and to all who played Knockout at the Bob and Joanne Kennedy family reunion, July 2003.

CONTENTS

● ●

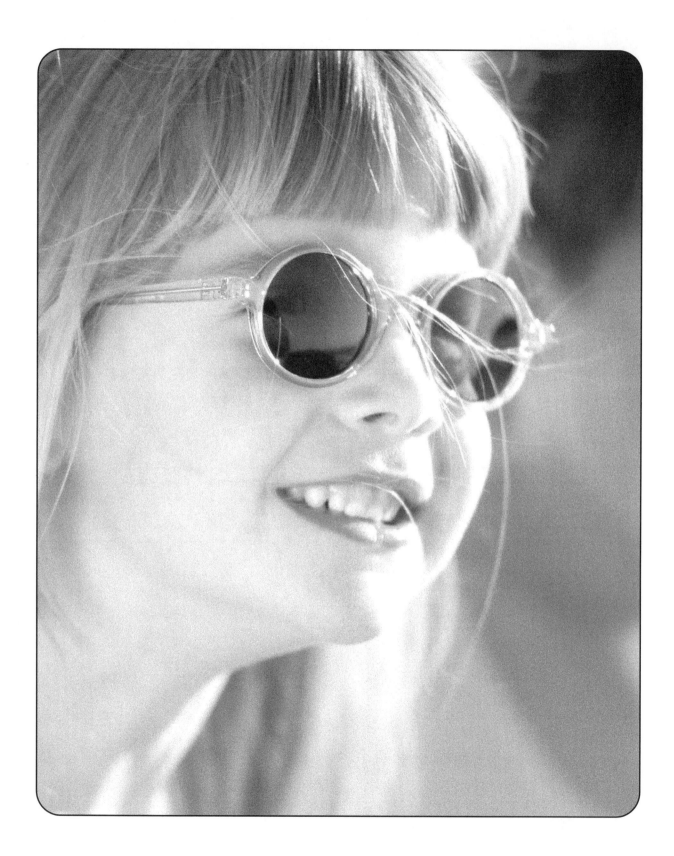

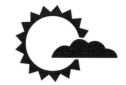

INTRODUCTION

There was most always a game going on Matoaka Court, the street where I lived as a child. We'd hustle to get out to the bus stop early so we could play "Red Light, Green Light" and "Mother, May I?" before bus number one rolled in. When we got home in the afternoon, we'd roam the woods or play kickball on the road, and when the fathers drove in from work in the early evening, they'd let us finish the play before we stepped to the curb to let their cars by.

There were only 12 houses or so in our small-town Williamsburg, Virginia, neighborhood, but at our baby boom peak in the late sixties and early seventies, there were more than 30 kids, and each house seemed to have a specialty. On the Varner's smooth concrete patio we'd play Kitty in the Corner. My own backyard was the place for badminton, and the Herrmann's driveway hosted countless games of H-O-R-S-E and Around the World—sometimes when the family's own kids were inside playing records.

And each game we played was forever stamped in my mind with "Matoaka Court" rules: My younger sister Amy and Kathy Varner got five strikes when we played softball instead of the usual three. In SPUD, you couldn't call the same person's number twice. No slamming in 4-Square or badminton. For the sake of being able to play at all, we learned how to set teams and juggle any game's details to accommodate groups that sometimes included a 7-year-old girl and a teenage boy who would go on to play minor league baseball, or nine kids who wanted to play and only one who could roll the ball over the kickball "plate."

On Friday nights in the summer our parents would let us play outside by streetlight for an extra hour—until the magic hour of 10 o'clock. We'd ride bikes in the street or play (I'm embarrassed to admit) a game called Cigarette Tag in the DeBord's spacious front yard. The object was to keep guessing cigarette brands until "It" said you had the right one, and then running like mad to get past the finish line on the other side without being tagged. Woe to you if you fell down or got tagged real hard— the DeBord's yard was also lined with horse chestnut trees and their prickly spines lay everywhere.

I'll never forget the thrill of waiting to be found in Sardines, a sort of reverse Hide and Seek game, listening to kids chat and call in the warm air, some of them walking right by my hiding spot in the dark.

Of course, idyllic times or not, we still had heated arguments and sometimes dirt clod fights. One time Doug McClennan left his front tooth in Johnny Byerly's back during a game of football. We never made it through a game of Kill the Guy with the Ball without at least one person going home crying, but mostly we had fun.

And that's the sole reason we played, to have fun. So it was interesting to attend the Matoaka Court Fourth of July reunion in 1998. Although all us former kids were now in our thirties and forties, everyone looked good. I had to laugh at the grown-up versions of people we'd considered "fat" as kids—all were fit and active and at the most 20 pounds overweight. Here we were, a living advertisement for the idea that active kids become active adults, and—I'd have to add after watching the kid's kids flock to the DeBord's yar for games of their own—active adults are more likely to have active offspring.

Unfortunately, we parents can't create Matoaka Courts in our kids' lives. Many kids don't have a pack of 30 playmates to run with after school. They aren't learning the rules for jump rope and Hopscotch during physical education class, because too often, they don't even have physical education and might never have recess. They have ballet and piano lessons on weeknights and play dates on Saturdays—not 7-hour softball games that start at daybreak and stop only for rain and for the pitcher to go to the grocery store with his mom. There are video games and computers and DVDs and any number of sedentary distractions. But most important of all these factors, in today's world few kids can roam unsupervised to "play."

And that's where you parents, and this book, come in. The games and fun that occurred naturally in our suburban and urban worlds of the sixties and seventies must be initiated these days by the only people who can bring together the know-how, resources, and motivation: Parents.

Need some motivation yourself, first? Consider these benefits of exercise:

✳ Reduce the risk of premature death
✳ Reduce the risk of developing and/or dying from heart disease
✳ Reduce high blood pressure or the risk of developing high blood pressure
✳ Reduce high cholesterol or the risk of developing high cholesterol
✳ Reduce the risk of developing colon cancer and breast cancer
✳ Reduce the risk of developing diabetes
✳ Reduce or maintain body weight or body fat
✳ Build and maintain healthy muscles, bones, and joints
✳ Reduce depression and anxiety
✳ Improve psychological well-being
✳ Enhanced work, recreation, and sport performance

The best part about physical activity is that it's an affordable luxury that any parent can give a child—money is no object when so many games can be played with just a tennis ball (or even a stick!).

POINTS FOR PARENTS

When trying to get your kids to be more active, keep in mind these three main points:

Don't mention weight. Overweight rates for adolescents doubled in the 1980s, and have since tripled; and overweight adolescents do have an increased health risk of everything from type 2 diabetes and heart disease to decreased mobility and physical endurance. Physical activity is a highly beneficial way to reduce your child's risk of obesity.

That said, no one wants to go out and run around because Mom says it will help them lose weight and "look so much better." In fact, any mention of "this will be good for you" will inevitably encourage resistance. Instead, get moving and stick with it and let the weight benefits take care of themselves.

Start small. I always laugh when I read the ongoing debate about how many times a week of sustained activity is enough to maintain your health... 20 minutes, 60 minutes, 10 times at 5 minutes each, etc., etc. The fact is that only 23 percent of American adults get enough leisure-time exercise to achieve cardiovascular fitness. In my book, any activity at all should be celebrated as a step in the right direction. (See the following pages for 20 non-game ways to add a little activity to your everyday life.)

If you think too hard, or too far down the line, it's all too easy to get intimidated and give up, as you might if you join a health club and overdo it the first day. Instead, start with a few easy games and try to remember to play them a few times one week. Later, increase your repertoire or the length of play. Or, you or your child may get interested in some other fitness training as the result of a game—

strength training for Crack the Whip (page 153, for example), or pitching practice for certain Stickball variations. The good things about fitness games, versus swimming laps or walking on the treadmill, is that even the youngest child will soon make the habit self-propelling. If she likes a game, in other words, she'll soon be reminding you that it's time to play—remember Candyland?

Make it a pleasure, not a punishment. Instead of replacing sedentary privileges, like computer time, with family fitness time, come up with extra time for fitness games, say, an extra hour on Saturdays instead of more chores, or one evening a week when you stay up a half-hour later so you can work in a game of flashlight tag. Even though you hope that eventually your kids will be playing more outdoor games and fewer video games, at the beginning it won't do to take away privileges if you want them to associate activity with fun and personal choice.

Make it fun for you, too. Even if you never swung a stickball bat or won a game of tag when you were a kid, you're the one who's going to hand this tradition down to your kids. So choose games you like, or would like to learn, so you can be genuinely enthusiastic about the idea. If you're an impatient person, take a look at the Super-Quick games listed in the chart on page 12.

When you can, join in. So many of these games need an adult around to balance the teams or make sure no one is downtrodden. If you can bear it, make time to join in the play, or at least the supervision, whenever you can. That sets a good example for the kids and tells them their activities are important to you—and hey, you'll be surprised how much exercise you can get in a kiddie game. Most important, even if they never lose a pound or make a shot, it will be time you've spent together in your children's growing years, and that time you can always treasure.

–Rose Kennedy

20 WAYS TO ADD ACTIVITY TO YOUR EVERYDAY LIFE

1. If you're going to shop or eat at the mall, go a half-hour before it opens and speed walk.

2. Instead of renting a video, go to a matinee at the theater.

3. Park far away from the store in the grocery store parking lot.

4. Park your cart in the middle of the grocery store and send individual family members to retrieve the groceries you need from faraway aisles—make a game of it.

5. Allow extra time in the morning to walk to the bus stop, rain or shine. Even if you go straight to work afterward, come back for the car.

6. Disconnect your automatic garage door opener.

7. Grow some vegetables or flowers.

8. Buy a clothesline and wash and air-dry at least a load a week.

9. Teach the kids how to change the sheets and make it a family ritual once a week.

10. Move the television at least two rooms from the kitchen.

11. Take trash directly to the outside bins instead of filling up a kitchen trash bag.

12. Start a compost bin or worm farm.

13. Instead of an ice cream treat at home, walk to the street vendor or local ice cream store.

14. On long trips, pack a lunch and eat and play catch at a rest area, not a fast-food restaurant.

15. Make a day of raking the yard by hand instead of using the leaf blower.

16. Turn off the air conditioner one day every summer weekend and use the sprinkler to cool off.

17. Wash the car together.

18. If one child has lessons or soccer practice, take supplies for a game to play with the ones who have to wait, instead of reading a magazine or book.

19. Make a loaf of homemade bread—no machine—once a week. It'll get better as you get more experienced, and you can use the rising time to check e-mails or go about your ordinary sedentary relaxation.

20. Rent a movie like *The Big Green* or *Bend It Like Beckham* and then spend an hour or two before or after learning the rules of the movie game, and playing.

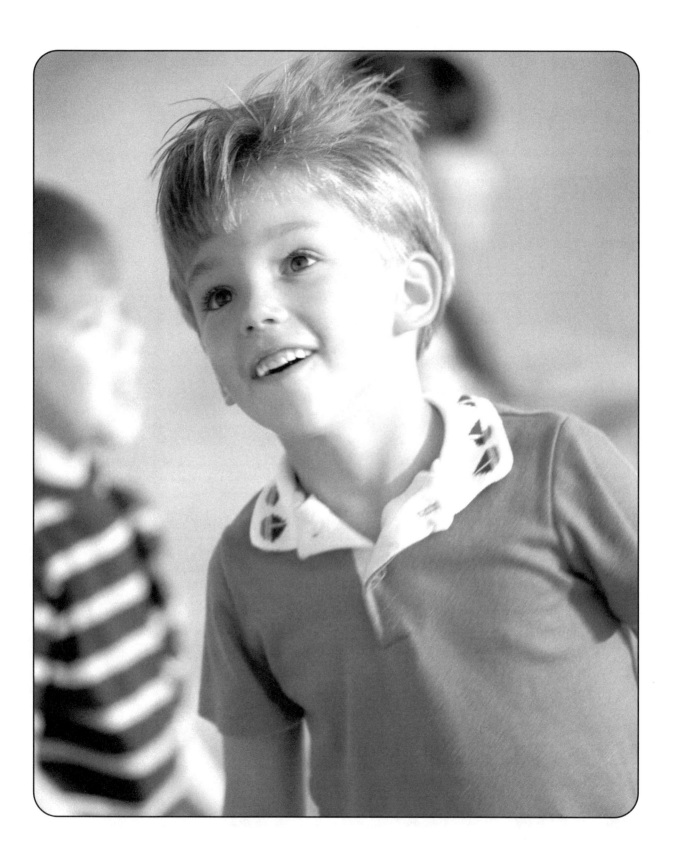

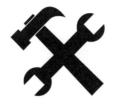

How to Use This Book

Lots of games are tantalizing, but to find the ones most likely to work with your group, start by considering the equipment required to play, and the weather, if you plan to be outside. Then consider the age of anyone who will be participating, and if the game offers fair ways for different ages to play together.

To assist you in the selection process, the games in this book are organized in three ways:

1. If you are searching for a specific game, take a look at the Index on page 176. You can search alphabetically by name.

2. If you don't have a specific activity in mind, but are interested in browsing several games that would work in different kinds of surroundings, the book itself is divided into chapters based upon location (for example, indoors, snow games, or city games). Each chapter begins with the simplest game and ends with the most difficult.

3. On the following pages is a chart with criteria to help you choose an appropriate game, from the numbers of players required to whether its best outdoors or in. It is sorted by age. See the box below for an explanation of the criteria.

PERFECT FOR PARTIES
These activities are loads of fun for all ages. Try playing several right in a row!

FUN FOR JUST ONE
These games only require one participant, although more are welcome.

HOURS OF FUN
Looking for a game to play for the entire afternoon? Try these hour-long activities.

NO EQUIPMENT NEEDED
The only equipment necessary for this game is tons of enthusiasm.

RAINY DAY FUN
Try these activities when you're trapped indoors.

FUN FOR THE WHOLE FAMILY
Planning a family reunion? Try these games that are fair for all ages.

SUPER-QUICK
These quick and easy activities can be completed in fifteen minutes or less.

BIG GROUP FUN
For large parties, try one of these activities, which need 6 or more participants.

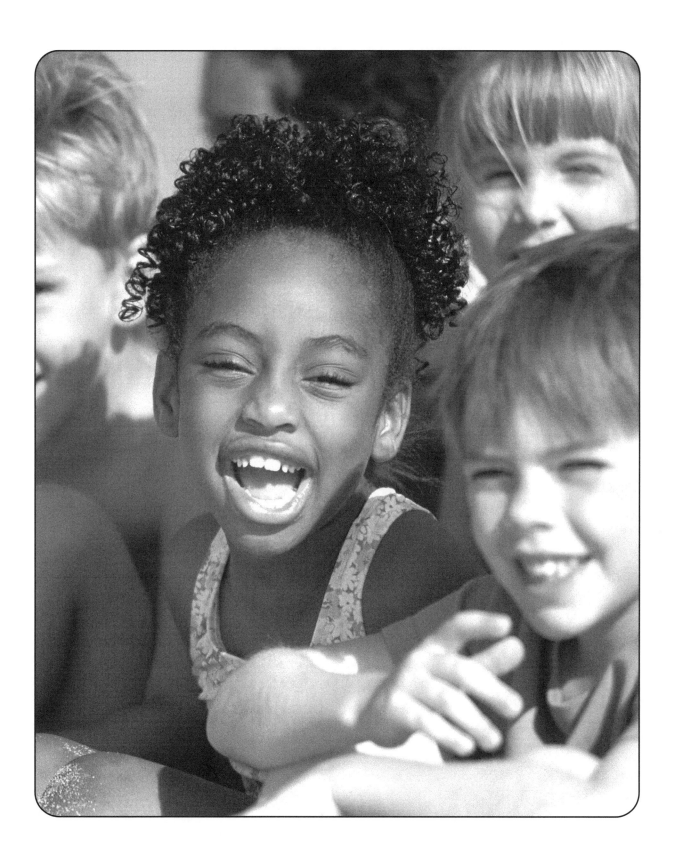

FAMILY FITNESS FUN GAME CHART

	LOCATION	AGE	INTENSITY LEVEL	PAGE #	WEATHER CONDITIONS	PARENTAL SUPERVISION
HOT POTATO	Indoor	3+	Easy	26	N/A	No
LONDON BRIDGE	Indoor	3+	Easy	28	N/A	No
WALK THE PLANK	Indoor	3+	Easy	30	N/A	No
SHOE HUSTLE	Indoor	3+	Easy	32	N/A	Yes
DIZZY BAT RACE	Outdoor	3+	Easy	68	Dry	No
SNOW HURDLES	Outdoor	3+	Active	142	Snow	Yes
ICE CUBE HUNT	Outdoor	3+	Moderate	144	Snow	Yes
FROZY TOESIES	Outdoor	3+	Moderate	158	Sun	Yes
BALLOON IN THE AIR	Indoor	4+	Easy	33	N/A	No
BUCKET BRIGADE	Outdoor	4+	Active	159	Sun	Yes
DROP THE CLOTHESPIN INTO A BOTTLE	Indoor	5+	Easy	34	N/A	No
BLINDFOLDED SHOE SHUFFLE	Indoor	5+	Easy	36	N/A	No
SIMON SAYS	Indoor	5+	Easy	37	N/A	No
BLINDMAN'S BLUFF	Indoor	5+	Easy	39	N/A	No
FOLLOW THE LEADER	Indoor	5+	Easy	41	N/A	No
LEAP FROG	Indoor	5+	Easy	43	N/A	No
BLINDFOLD FOUR CORNER	Indoor	5+	Easy	45	N/A	No
STONE TEACHER	Indoor	5+	Easy	47	N/A	No
FRUIT BASKET	Indoor	5+	Easy	49	N/A	Yes
POP BOTTLE RING TOSS	Outdoor	5+	Easy	70	Dry	No
RED LIGHT, GREEN LIGHT	Outdoor	5+	Easy	72	Dry	No
FIVE DOLLARS	Outdoor	5+	Moderate	74	Dry	No
CAT AND MOUSE	Outdoor	5+	Moderate	76	Dry	No
MOTHER MAY I	Outdoor	5+	Easy	78	Dry	No
QUEENIE	Outdoor	5+	Easy	80	Dry	No

PERFECT FOR PARTIES	FUN FOR JUST ONE	HOURS OF FUN	NO EQUIPMENT NEEDEED	RAINY DAY FUN	FUN FOR THE WHOLE FAMILY	SUPER-QUICK	BIG GROUP FUN
★				★		★	
			★	★			
★					★		
★						★	
★		★			★		★
★		★			★		★
★						★	
★				★		★	
							★
★	★			★		★	
★							
			★			★	
★							★
			★	★			
			★				
★						★	
				★			
★					★		★
★	★				★	★	
			★			★	
					★		★
★			★			★	★
★			★				
★						★	

FAMILY FITNESS FUN
GAME CHART

	LOCATION	AGE	INTENSITY LEVEL	PAGE #	WEATHER CONDITIONS	PARENTAL SUPERVISION
WHEELBARROW RACE	Outdoor	5+	Easy	82	Dry	No
SNOW TAG	Outdoor	5+	Active	146	Snow	Yes
JUMP ROPE	Outdoor	5+	Active	121	Dry	No
HIT THE STICK	Outdoor	5+	Easy	124	Dry	No
HOPSCOTCH	Both	5+	Moderate	126	Dry	No
BASIC TAG	Outdoor	5+	Active	106	Warm	No
SHADOW TAG	Outdoor	5+	Active	111	Sun	No
BODY TAG	Outdoor	5+	Active	109	Warm	No
CHAIN TAG	Outdoor	5+	Active	109	Warm	No
CLOTHESPIN TAG	Outdoor	5+	Active	110	Warm	No
ELBOW TAG	Outdoor	5+	Active	110	Warm	No
FLOUR TAG	Outdoor	5+	Active	110	Warm	No
TURTLE TAG	Outdoor	5+	Active	111	Warm	No
BLOB TAG	Outdoor	5+	Moderate	112	Dry	Yes
BANDAID TAG	Outdoor	5+	Active	113	Dry	No
MARCO POLO	Outdoor	5+	Easy	161	Sun	Yes
BLIND FETCH	Indoor	6+	Moderate	51	N/A	Yes
SNEAKY PATTY	Indoor	6+	Moderate	53	N/A	Yes
BASIC RELAY	Outdoor	6+	Moderate	84	Dry	Yes
TRASH TARGET	Outdoor	6+	Active	163	Sun	Yes
HOPPING H$_2$O	Outdoor	6+	Moderate	165	Sun	Yes
CLOSE SHAVE SHOOTOUT	Outdoor	6+	Moderate	166	Sun	Yes
WET T-SHIRT RELAY	Outdoor	6+	Active	168	Sun	Yes
HIDE AND SEEK	Indoor	7+	Moderate	55	N/A	No

PERFECT FOR PARTIES	FUN FOR JUST ONE	HOURS OF FUN	NO EQUIPMENT NEEDED	RAINY DAY FUN	FUN FOR THE WHOLE FAMILY	SUPER-QUICK	BIG GROUP FUN
	★		★		★	★	★
	★				★	★	
	★						
		★					
			★				
			★				
			★				
			★				
			★				
			★				
			★				
			★				
			★				
★			★				
		★			★		★
★				★			
★							★
							★
					★		
★					★		★
★					★	★	
★			★		★		★

FAMILY FITNESS FUN GAME CHART

	LOCATION	AGE	INTENSITY LEVEL	PAGE #	WEATHER CONDITIONS	PARENTAL SUPER...
INDOOR BALLOON RACE	Indoor	7+	Easy	58	N/A	No
LIMBO	Indoor	7+	Moderate	60	N/A	No
CAPTURE THE FLAG	Outdoor	7+	Active	89	Dry	No
STEAL THE BACON	Outdoor	7+	Active	91	Dry	No
DODGEBALL	Outdoor	7+	Active	94	Dry	Yes
TEN AGAIN	Outdoor	7+	Active	100	Dry	No
RED ROVER	Outdoor	7+	Active	101	Dry	Yes
SHARE-A-PAIR RACE	Outdoor	7+	Active	103	Dry	No
ICE AGE TUG-OF-WAR	Outdoor	7+	Active	148	Snow	Yes
GARAGE VOLLEYBALL	Outdoor	7+	Moderate	130	Dry	No
BOX BALL	Outdoor	7+	Moderate	131	Dry	No
SLOW-PITCH STICKBALL	Outdoor	7+	Active	132	Dry	Yes
FAST-PITCH STICKBALL	Outdoor	7+	Active	136	Dry	Yes
FUNGO STICKBALL	Outdoor	7+	Active	138	Dry	Yes
FLASHLIGHT TAG	Outdoor	7+	Active	116	Night	No
BLINDFOLD TAG	Outdoor	7+	Active	116	Dry	No
BROOM TAG	Outdoor	7+	Active	116	Dry	No
FREEZE TAG	Outdoor	7+	Active	117	Warm	No
TV TAG	Outdoor	7+	Active	117	Dry	No
CONKERS	Indoor	8+	Easy	62	N/A	Yes
SLEDDING SNOW TARGET	Outdoor	8+	Active	150	Snow	Yes
TWINS	Outdoor	8+	Active	152	Snow	No
CRACK THE WHIP	Outdoor	9+	Active	153	Snow	No

	PERFECT FOR PARTIES	FUN FOR JUST ONE	HOURS OF FUN	NO EQUIPMENT NEEDED	RAINY DAY FUN	FUN FOR THE WHOLE FAMILY	SUPER-QUICK	BIG GROUP FUN
	★				★			★
					★	★		★
								★
								★
								★
			★					
	★			★				★
	★							
	★							
			★			★		
			★					
			★			★		★
	★		★			★		★
			★			★		★
				★				
				★				
			★					
						★		★
				★				
	★			★				

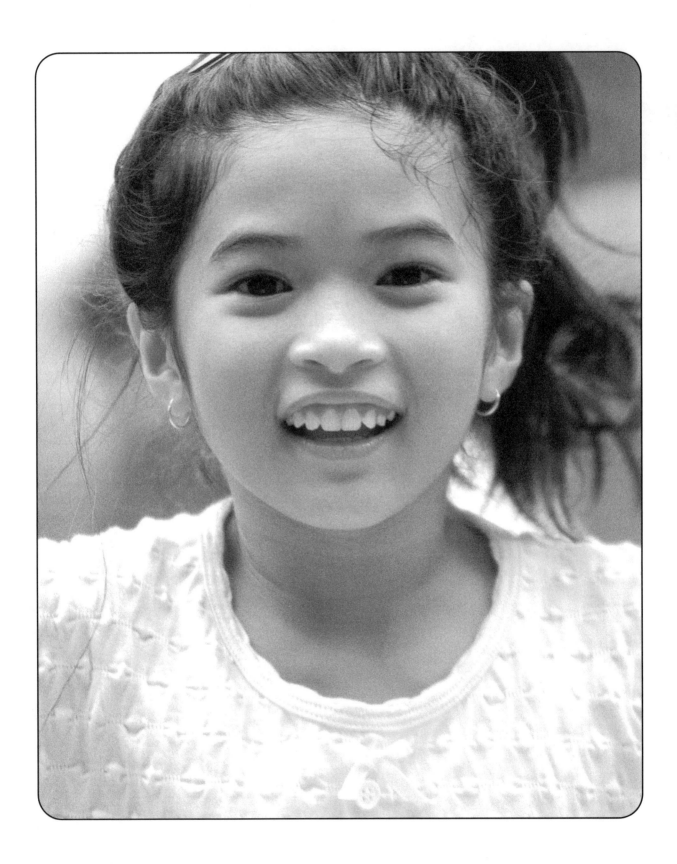

1

ALWAYS ACTIVE

Add aerobic benefits to games without taking away the fun

Among other fitness goals, the President's Council on Physical Fitness recommends at least three 20-minute bouts of continuous aerobic rhythmic exercise each week for the average, healthy person. Of course, most of us get nowhere near that much, nor do our kids. But the thought of jogging or taking an aerobics class can be daunting.

Ever consider games instead? Certain brisk competitions will certainly raise heart rates to the recommended levels—and if the group is having fun, no one is going to notice that they're playing longer and harder each time. Adults over 35 should check with their doctor first, and everyone should warm up with a few stretches and carry plenty of water. Then, get moving. It's the fun way to physical fitness.

MEASURING YOUR HEART RATE

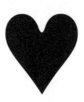 Heart rate is widely accepted as a good method for measuring intensity during running, swimming, cycling, and other aerobic activities. Exercise that doesn't raise your heart rate to a certain level and keep it there for at least 20 minutes won't contribute significantly to cardiovascular fitness.

The heart rate adults should maintain is called your Target Heart Rate. There are several ways of figuring out what your appropriate target heart rate is. First, you figure out your maximum heart rate, which is the number you get when you subtract your age from the number 220. Your target heart rate is 70 percent of your maximum heart rate. So, the simplest formula for target heart rate is this:

MAXIMUM HEART RATE (220 – AGE) X 0.7
For example, the Maximum Heart Rate for a 40-year-old would be 180.
$(220 - 40 = 180)$

Therefore, the Target Heart Rate for a 40-year old would be 126.
$(180 \times 0.7 = 126)$

Some methods for figuring the target rate take individual levels of fitness into consideration. Here is one of them, called the Karvonen Method.

As a parent, one of the most important things you can do for your children's health and positive outlook is to give them a positive introduction to activities and games. If you do this while they're young, starting as toddlers, they'll carry the idea that they're "participators" into their adolescent and teen years.

Of course, you don't want to push too hard or too fast. Find something your young child truly enjoys, and try not to mind if they

1. Determine your Maximum Heart Rate.

2. Determine your Resting Heart Rate. This is pulse rate you maintain while you are sitting quietly or sleeping. You can find this by taking your pulse after sitting quietly or lying down for at least 5 minutes.

3. Subtract your Resting Heart Rate from your Maximum Heart Rate to determine Heart Rate Reserve.

4. Take 70 percent of your Heart Rate Reserve is your Heart Rate Raise.

5. Add the Heart Rate Raise to your Resting Heart Rate to find your Target Rate.

When checking your heart rate during a workout, take your pulse within 5 seconds of interrupting exercise because your pulse can decrease dramatically once you stop moving. Count your pulse for 10 seconds and multiply by six to get the per-minute rate.

Note: These formulas are not applicable to children. The maximum heart rate in healthy children is about 200 beats per minute. According to the American Heart Association, there is no need to arbitrarily restrict healthy children to lower heart rates.

Source: President's Council on Physical Fitness and Sports

don't stick to the rules, as long as they're running around. Most important, get in there and play with them! The whole family will reap health benefits while bonding and having fun together. And that doesn't happen if your child plays with the beach ball only at day care, or knows mom is the one who always watches from the lounge chair, coffee in hand. Don't make your child beg you to play with her!

Faced with a large crowd of different interests and ages, you may be tempted to pour a glass of wine and get out the DVD player, but it's actually the best time to get everyone involved in some large-scale family fitness games.

There are bound to be a few in the group who know what they're doing, and they can initiate the others. Plus, a bit of exercise will improve attitudes and keep everyone too busy to start the ordinary arguments.

More important than those conveniences, though, is giving the whole concept of outdoor activity a positive spin with your kids. If they have fun in a big group, they're more likely to try the same game again another time with a few friends or siblings. They may even wheedle you into being more active with just the family, too!

Do you remember when the summer evenings were long and you'd play in the neighborhood until the last possible minute, running and calling and hiding and throwing? Or endless afternoons spent "hanging out" with friends on the stoop or in the park, batting a ball, drawing a Hopscotch board? Make sure your kids spend some time like that, just being kids, with these classic games that every child should know.

And if you've never played any of them, or didn't have the idyllic childhood we described? Remedy that by learning these games alongside your kids, and you'll all have a legacy to pass along to the next generation together.

CHOOSING TEAMS

As the "adult in charge" of games, you should take responsibility for making sure teams are somewhat even. Here are a number of ways to pick teams. If you're smart, you'll quickly review who will end up on each team in your head before announcing how you'll determine who's on which side (or sides).

It's usually a bad idea to have captains pick sides—it's just an invitation for spite and hurt feelings, even among ordinarily mature kids or adults. Instead, divide teams along lines of:

❊ Biggest shoe sizes against smallest
❊ Birth month, starting with January
❊ Eye color
❊ First name alphabetically
❊ Hair color
❊ Last name alphabetically
❊ Likes root beer, loathes root beer
❊ Long hair against short
❊ Long sleeves against short sleeves
❊ Oldest—youngest, next oldest—next youngest, and so forth
❊ Painted fingernails versus not
❊ People who traveled the farthest against people who live the closest
❊ Tallest—shortest on one team, next tallest—next shortest on the other, and so forth
❊ White socks versus colored
❊ Who can hold their breath the longest, who lets their breath out first on one team, who can hold their breath the second longest, who lets their breath out second on the other, and so forth

In most games, you can also use one of these variations to determine who's It next, instead of basing it on performance in the game.

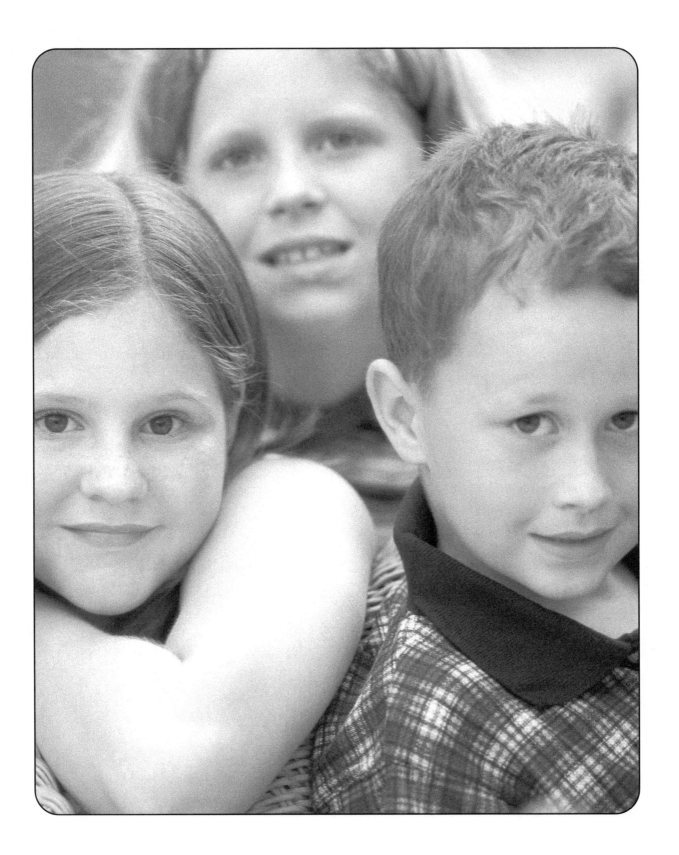

2

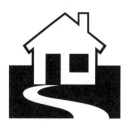

INDOOR GAMES

In decades past, "indoors" was the place you had to stay when you had the measles or the weather was foul, a la The Cat in the Hat. Today, the great indoors is an all-too-comfortable spot to hang out day in and day out. To change gears and combat boredom, next time a group comes over and plops in front of the DVD player, rev up the atmosphere with some active games. Some of these are appropriate for even the youngest kids, so keep them in mind for playdates and parties—and don't forget to share some ideas with your day care or after-school program. To make it convenient, keep a space in the house fairly clear, even if it's just the basement. Also keep supplies for some of the simpler games assembled and at the ready in shoe boxes. The idea is to have fun and get moving around, and when you've worked up to the point where "games" seem more like roughhousing, move it outside!

Hot Potato

This is one of those fun games that you probably played in kindergarten. It's a timeless classic. The excitement builds as the potato gets passed from hand to hand, with everyone wondering when exactly the music will stop. This is a game that parents can enjoy right along with the kids.

How to Play

* When you start the musical selection of your choice, the players begin to pass a raw potato around.
* When you stop the music, the one holding the potato is out.
* The last player remaining wins.

To be fair, whoever plays the music should face away from the game so they can't see who has the potato before they decide to stop the music.

What You Need

* Enough space for all the players to sit in a circle.
* Raw potato (or a ball)
* Stereo or boom box to play music

Setting Up

Have all the players sit in a circle in an area where they can easily hear the music you'll play.

PERFECT FOR PARTIES

RAINY DAY FUN

SUPER-QUICK

INDOOR OR OUTDOOR:
Both

AGES:
3 and older

HOW MANY CAN PLAY?
3 or more

WEATHER:
If outside,
warm and dry

TIME REQUIRED:
At least 2 minutes

**PARENTAL SUPERVISION/
INVOLVEMENT:**
Not necessary

INTENSITY LEVEL:
Super Easy

PASS THE PRESENT

Pass the Present is a fun variation of Hot Potato—and a birthday party and shower favorite. To play, wrap a small gift in at least seven layers of wrapping paper. Whoever is holding the present when the music stops unwraps just one layer of wrapping paper. If it doesn't reveal the gift, he's out and the game proceeds. But whoever is holding the present when the last layer of wrapping is removed gets to keep it.

London Bridge

A must for the first birthday party of social awareness, say at age 5 or so, London Bridge can also be everyday fun. Just make sure you have an adult or two on hand to corral the kids, sing the loudest until some of the youngsters know the words, and to break if up if the London Bridge keeps coming down aggressively on slower players.

What You Need

No equipment needed.

Setting Up

Two players face each other and form a "bridge" by raising their arms up over their heads, leaning forward, and joining hands.

How to Play

* Players hold hands and pass under the bridge one at a time in a continuous circle while singing, "London Bridge is falling down, falling down, falling down. London Bridge is falling down, my fair lady."
* On the last word of the song, the two players comprising the bridge bring their arms down and trap the player who was passing through at that moment.

NO EQUIPMENT NEEDED

RAINY DAY FUN

INDOOR OR OUTDOOR:
Both

AGES:
3 and older

HOW MANY CAN PLAY?
8 or more

WEATHER:
If outside, warm and dry

TIME REQUIRED:
At least 2 minutes

PARENTAL SUPERVISION/ INVOLVEMENT:
Not necessary

INTENSITY LEVEL:
Super Easy

✳ When a player is caught, the group sings: "Take the key and lock him up, lock him up, lock him up. Take the key and lock him up, my fair lady."

✳ The player who is caught is eliminated, and play continues until one player remains.

RULES OF PLAY

✳ If the bridge comes down and no one is caught, the round is repeated without any players being eliminated.

✳ A new pair of players is selected to be the bridge after each round of play.

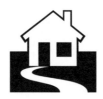

Walk the Plank

Ahoy, mateys. You all know who makes you walk a plank. What you may not know is that practice with a game such as this improves your child's balance, which in turn can improve his posture, strengthen his back, and make him less prone to injury during sports activities. But who cares about all that when you get a chance to get your hands on the household binoculars... with permission!

What You Need

✳ Twenty-foot length of rope or masking tape
✳ Binoculars

Setting Up

✳ This game can be played on soft grass, pavement, or indoors on wooden floors or linoleum.
✳ Lay out a 20-foot long rope (or 20 feet of tape) in a straight line.

How to Play

✳ Players take turns looking through the binoculars the wrong way while trying to walk the length of the rope.
✳ The player who makes it to the end of the plank first is the winner.

Rules of Play

✳ Players get two chances to make it to end of the plank during each turn.

✳ If a player steps off the plank he must start from the beginning; if he steps off the plank a second time, he is disqualified.

✳ If no players make it all the way to the end of the plank, the player who made it farthest is the winner.

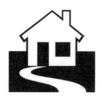

Shoe Hustle

If your preschooler is among the proud people who know how to tie shoes, have we got a game for you! This is simple and fun, and you can do it at the end of the day with the family, or at any picnic or birthday party—just as long as everyone's wearing shoes that tie, and none of them are too smelly!

What You Need

Enough space for everyone to sit in a circle on the floor or on a blanket in the grass or sand.

How to Play

* Everyone sits in a circle on the floor or blanket to remove their shoes. Then each person takes the shoestrings out of their shoes and tucks them inside.
* Pile everyone's shoes in the center of the circle.
* Have a responsible adult shuffle them a bit, and then everyone moves two spaces to the right in the circle.
* At the "Go!" signal, everyone races for the pile, finds his shoes, laces them up, and puts them on.
* The first one finished and standing up is the winner!

Tips for Making It Fair

If adults or older kids are playing, mix their socks and unlaced shoestrings in with the shoes, so they have to sort through the pile to find all of the above instead of just two shoes, which should even things out a bit.

PERFECT FOR PARTIES

SUPER-QUICK

INDOOR OR OUTDOOR:
Both

AGES:
3 and older

HOW MANY CAN PLAY?
Up to 5 little ones, up to 8 with a mixed age group

WEATHER:
If outside, warm and dry

TIME REQUIRED:
At least 10 minutes

PARENTAL SUPERVISION/ INVOLVEMENT:
Yes, the first time

INTENSITY LEVEL:
Super Easy

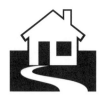

Balloon in the Air

Keeping a balloon in the air causes chaos on the ground—and it's just this mad kind of running around that the pre-school set adores. It's also a great game if you have older kids wanting to play and little ones begging to be part of the action. Just pair a bigger, taller kid with a pre-schooler, and play two-person teams so everyone is included in the fun.

What You Need

❋ One non-helium balloon for each player, plus a few extras.

Setting Up

❋ Blow up the balloons and tie them off. Give one balloon to each child, and place them in an area where they can move around freely, like the back yard or a 10-foot by 10-foot carpeted floor.

How to Play

❋ On the "go" signal, each child tosses her balloon into the air and then does whatever she can to try to keep it from hitting the ground—without catching or holding it.
❋ Whoever keeps their balloon up the longest wins.

FEATHER IN THE AIR

For this variation, give each child a feather to keep aloft—just by blowing, no hands allowed. Whoever has the longest "flight" wins.

PERFECT FOR PARTIES

RAINY DAY FUN

SUPER-QUICK

INDOOR OR OUTDOOR:
Both

AGES:
4 and older

HOW MANY CAN PLAY?
2 or more

WEATHER:
If outside, warm and dry

TIME REQUIRED:
At least 5 minutes

PARENTAL SUPERVISION/ INVOLVEMENT:
Not necessary, but fun

INTENSITY LEVEL:
Easy

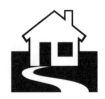

Drop the Clothespin into a Bottle

Although this is a traditional favorite at children's birthday parties, you can also play with just one, and you'll really get much better the more you practice. Parents can wow the kids by practicing in secret after they've gone to bed, and then one day revealing their newfound skill.

WHAT YOU NEED

* Clean dry coffee can with plastic lid
* Ten to 20 plastic or wooden clothespins

GIVE THE GAME A THEME

If you're having a theme party, make sure to decorate the canister and draw on the clothespins accordingly. Then change the name of the game. For example, play "drop the lava into the volcano" for a Hawaiian theme, or "drop the Dursleys into the Secret Chamber" for a Harry Potter party.

SETTING UP

Cut a hole in the center of a plastic coffee can lid and place the lid on the can. Start with a 1-inch hole, and then see if anyone can drop a clothespin through the hole from a standing position. If not, keep increasing the size of the hole until it's skill-appropriate. You can also make several canisters with graduated hole sizes.

PERFECT FOR PARTIES

RAINY DAY FUN

FUN FOR JUST ONE

SUPER-QUICK

INDOOR OR OUTDOOR:
Both

AGES:
5 and older

HOW MANY CAN PLAY?
Any number, including 1

WEATHER:
Any

TIME REQUIRED:
5 to 10 minutes per try

PARENTAL SUPERVISION/ INVOLVEMENT:
Not necessary, but this is a good one for adults to try

INTENSITY LEVEL:
Super Easy

How to Play

* Give each player five clothespins.
* Taking turns, each player stands over the canister, straddling his feet on either side, and tries to drop the clothespins through the hole into the canister.

Rules of Play

* Whoever gets the most clothespins in the can wins the round.
* If you play several rounds, you may keep a tally of total pins "scored" or total rounds won to determine a winner.
* Players may not bend or stoop while tossing clothespins, but they may hunch their shoulders over and look down.

Tip for the players

To take better aim, close one eye before tossing—it helps your depth perception.

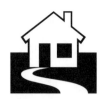

Blindfolded Shoe Shuffle

We found this game on a website called www.funattic.com. It was submitted to the site by a man identified only as "Mr. Minty." It's a great party game, or you can play with your own kids to break the fatigue at the end of a long day (when everyone's shoes are probably already off anyway.) For the very young, like age 3, it's got an educational angle, because it's a fun way to learn to sort and categorize. Thanks, Mr. Minty!

HOW TO PLAY

✳ The referee jumbles all the shoes and then shouts, "Go!"
✳ The first person to find his or her shoes by touch and smell alone and put them on is the winner.

WHAT YOU NEED

✳ Blindfold for each player
✳ A pair of tie-up shoes for each player

SETTING UP

✳ Each person puts on a blindfold and takes off his or her shoes.
✳ Throw the shoes into a pile in the middle of the floor (or the middle of a marked off area on soft grass).
✳ Designate one observer as the referee.

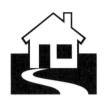

Simon Says

There was a bubblegum pop hit by this name in 1968. It had the refrain, "Do it when Simon says... And you will never be out." And that's pretty much how it is. About anyone can have fun playing Simon Says, toddlers to teenagers, and you can start and finish while you wait on the bus or play several rounds while a load of laundry is drying.

WHAT YOU NEED

No equipment needed.

SETTING UP

Players can stand in a circle or in a straight line facing the Leader. All players must be able to see the Leader from where they stand.

HOW TO PLAY

❋ The Leader makes gestures while giving instructions that start with the phrase "Simon Says."

❋ Any players who don't do what "Simon Says" are disqualified, as are those who follow instructions that were not preceded by the phrase "Simon Says." For example, the Leader bends over to touch his toes while saying, "Simon Says touch your toes," and then quickly says, "Touch your knees." Any players who are touching

NO EQUIPMENT NEEDED

SUPER-QUICK

INDOOR OR OUTDOOR:
Both

AGES:
5 and older

HOW MANY CAN PLAY?
3 or more

WEATHER:
If outside, no wet grass

TIME REQUIRED:
At least 10 minutes

PARENTAL SUPERVISION/ INVOLVEMENT:
Not necessary

INTENSITY LEVEL:
Easy

their knees are disqualified because the Leader did not say, "Simon Says touch your knees."

✳ Play continues with the Leader making gestures and giving instructions until only one player remains. This player becomes the new Leader.

TIPS FOR THE LEADER

There are several ways to fool the other players when it's your turn to be the Leader. Try adding a speed element to the game by giving instructions very quickly—anyone who can't keep up is out. Also, you can confuse the other players by telling them to do one thing while showing them a completely different gesture. For example, say "Simon Says touch your nose with your left hand" while touching your ear with your right hand.

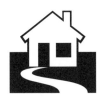

Blindman's Bluff

Charles Dickens described the street urchins playing Blindman's Bluff in *A Christmas Carol*, and the game probably dates back to the ancient Romans. Part of the appeal is its simplicity: There's not much needed beyond a group of exuberant players and a trustworthy blindfold. To be authentic, make a tradition of playing at Christmas, and any other time of year when the family or neighborhood kids gather—and can stand still long enough to tie a bit of bandana about their eyes.

WHAT YOU NEED

❋ A blindfold, shirt, or piece of cloth that can be used to cover It's eyes.

SETTING UP

❋ The player chosen as It is blindfolded.

HOW TO PLAY

❋ Players spin It (who has been blindfolded) around three times, quickly form a circle, join hands, and start skipping counterclockwise.
❋ Players continue skipping until it calls "Stop," and then freeze in place. It points, and the person closest to his finger enters the circle.

PERFECT FOR PARTIES

BIG GROUP FUN

INDOOR OR OUTDOOR:
Both

AGES:
5 and older

HOW MANY CAN PLAY?
8 or more

WEATHER:
If outside, warm and dry

TIME REQUIRED:
At least 20 minutes

PARENTAL SUPERVISION/ INVOLVEMENT:
Not necessary

INTENSITY LEVEL:
Easy

✳ It, who is still blindfolded, chases the player inside the circle until she is caught, or until 2 minutes have passed. If tagged, It tries to identify the player by touching her face.

✳ If It guesses the player's identity, they switch places for the next round of play.

BLINDMAN'S TAG

In this variation, players do not stand in a circle. Instead, after spinning It around three times they scatter over the playing field. It must then try to tag someone and guess her identity. Because It is blindfolded, players are encouraged to yell, scream, and otherwise taunt It to help orient him. As in Blindman's Buff, if It tags a player and guesses her identity they switch places for the next round.

Follow the Leader

Ever since the Disney musical, we'll always picture Peter Pan at the head of any Follow the Leader game. Rediscover how fun it can be with a few popular adults leading the first couple of rounds. This game also emphasizes the strength of diversity. So what if a kid isn't the best catcher on the team? In Follow the Leader he can show off his whistling, skipping, or crouching skills... everybody's good at something.

WHAT YOU NEED

No equipment needed.

SETTING UP

❋ Players stand in a straight line behind the Leader.

HOW TO PLAY

❋ The Leader makes movements, gestures, and sounds that other players must mimic.
❋ The Leader should always be moving (walking, skipping, jumping, and so on) to keep other players on their toes.

NO EQUIPMENT NEEDED

RAINY DAY FUN

INDOOR OR OUTDOOR:
Both

AGES:
5 and older

HOW MANY CAN PLAY?
4 or more

WEATHER:
If outside, warm and dry

TIME REQUIRED:
At least 10 minutes for each round

PARENTAL SUPERVISION/ INVOLVEMENT:
Not necessary

INTENSITY LEVEL:
Easy

Rules of Play

✳ Players who don't imitate the Leader correctly are disqualified.

✳ Players who can't keep up with the moving line are out.

✳ Choose a new Leader every 5 to 10 minutes to keep the game exciting.

FOLLOW THE LEADER... INTO THE WATER

In a version of Follow the Leader we call Walk the Plank, the leader walks down the diving board and then does any flaky or funny dive (or belly flop) he likes. After he swims to the side and gets out, the next player tries to follow his example. The results are hilarious! Note: Only one player should be on the diving board or in the water below the board at a time.

Be a Funny Leader

Make your movements as silly as you can. Try combining a simple gesture, like tugging your ear, with singing a song, like Mary had a Little lamb, in a high and squeaky voice.

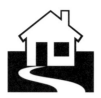

Leap Frog

Little kids are always jumping around anyway. Make this activity even more fun with a few rounds of Leap Frog. If the youngest players can't quite "get" the concept, start with just jumping around like frogs and saying "ribbit." And make sure that no one's wearing boots, heavy shoes, or metal belt buckles that will clomp another little froggie in the head.

What You Need

No equipment needed

Setting Up

✳ Players crouch on the floor in a single-file row with about three feet between players, facing forward. Players should be on their knees with their heads covered by their hands.

How to Play

✳ The last player in line stands up and jumps over each other player one at a time.
✳ The jumper puts his hands on another person's back and pushes off to propel himself forward.

NO EQUIPMENT NEEDED

INDOOR OR OUTDOOR:
Both

AGES:
5 and older

HOW MANY CAN PLAY?
3 or more

WEATHER:
If outside, warm and dry

TIME REQUIRED:
At least 20 minutes

PARENTAL SUPERVISION/ INVOLVEMENT:
Not necessary, but fun

INTENSITY LEVEL:
Easy

RULES OF PLAY

When the jumper finishes leaping over all the players, he crouches at the head of the line, and the player in the back of the line gets a turn to leap.

FROG RACE

If there are at least eight players, Leap Frog can become a racing game. Players are divided equally into teams of at least four. The number of teams depends on the number of players. Each team crouches on the floor to form its own line. A person who isn't part of the game yells, "On your mark. Get set. Go!" The player at the end of each line stands and leaps over his teammates. When the player reaches the front of line, he or she crouches down and yells "Go," at which point the next player in line starts leaping. The team whose players jump fastest is the winner. In another variation, a starting line and stopping line are designated, and the first team to "leap frog" across the finish line is the winner.

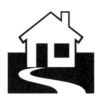

Blindfold
Four Corner

This is a quick game that's perfect for club meetings, slumber parties, indoor recess, or any time a group is gathered at your house and you want to be active—not clustered around the video games. Still, you're not making a big time commitment, here. You can play one round in 10 minutes, or play for hours with a few die-hards, depending on how long everyone stays interested.

WHAT YOU NEED

✳ Blindfold

SETTING UP

✳ Clear a corridor at least 3 feet wide around the perimeter of the room. Secure any breakables.
✳ Place a chair in the middle.
✳ Select one player to wear a blindfold and sit in the chair.

HOW TO PLAY

✳ Once the blindfolded player is in position, the other players must move quietly into to stand still in one of the four corners. They have 10 seconds.

PERFECT FOR PARTIES

SUPER-QUICK

INDOOR OR OUTDOOR:
Indoors

AGES:
5 and older

HOW MANY CAN PLAY?
6 or more

TIME REQUIRED:
10 minutes per one round, at the most

PARENTAL SUPERVISION/ INVOLVEMENT:
Not necessary, but fun

INTENSITY LEVEL:
Easy

* The blindfolded player counts out loud to 10. When he's done, all the others must be still and in one of the corners.
* The blindfolded player points to one of the corners and all the players in that corner are out of the game.

RULES OF PLAY

* If a player is not in a corner by the time the blindfolded player finishes counting, that player is out.
* To be fair, you're not allowed to make noises in one corner and then quickly move to another. If you do, you're out.
* If no one is in a selected corner, all the players have 5 seconds to get to another corner before the blindfolded player selects a new corner.
* When three or fewer people are left, only two can be in the same corner.
* When two people are left, each must choose a different corner.
* The last person found becomes the new blindfolded player.

ELBOW-POINTING VARIATION

So that the person blindfolded in the middle has to stay alert, make a rule that he or she can only point to his chosen corner with his elbow. If he fails, and at least one of the players realizes and calls, "Norton," the players in that corner are safe after all.

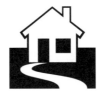

Stone Teacher

Ever notice how much kids love to play school, even the ones who have never been? This game introduces the concept of following instructions from a leader and trying to get ahead of others, but it's not like a young child's hearing, "Ha ha! You lose!" because no one has to leave the game.

How to Play

✳ The stone teacher hides her hands behind her back while she decides which hand to hide the stone in.

✳ Then she brings her hands forward with closed fists and lets the first player choose which of the teacher's hands she thinks the stone is in. If the player is correct, she moves down one step. If not, she stays on the same step.

✳ Then the teacher again hides her hands behind her back, and the next player gets to choose.

✳ The first person to the bottom step is the winner and the new stone teacher.

RAINY DAY FUN

INDOOR OR OUTDOOR:
Both

AGES:
5 and older

HOW MANY CAN PLAY?
3 or fewer if indoors,
4 to 5 if outdoors

WEATHER:
If outside, warm and
dry

TIME REQUIRED:
At least 20 minutes

**PARENTAL SUPERVISION/
INVOLVEMENT:**
Yes, or at least a
responsible preteen

INTENSITY LEVEL:
Easy

WHAT YOU NEED

✳ Safe stairs, at least 6 feet wide if you're outdoors. If indoors, the stairs should be carpeted and all the same height from riser to riser.

✳ A small stone

SETTING UP

Have all players sit at the top of the stairs. Designate the adult as the stone teacher (at least the first time) and give her the stone.

Fruit Basket

Like musical chairs without the music, this is a perfect birthday party game. You can play it anywhere, even poolside with lawn chairs, because it requires only chairs to sit on and an adult to supervise. It's also great as an ice-breaker at all-ages parties or big family reunions, because players have to observe the other players' physical attributes carefully, or learn something else about them.

Setting Up

❋ Place chairs in a circle on the driveway, in the yard or in the dining room. You need one fewer chair than there are players.

How to Play

❋ Everyone sits in a chair, except the person selected to be the caller for the first round. He or she makes a remark that describes at least two players in the group, such as, "I'm grateful for people with blue eyes." Everyone with blue eyes stands and changes places.
❋ While everyone's scurrying for a chair, a parent takes one away.
❋ The person left standing is out.
❋ The caller then makes a remark such as, "I'm grateful for everyone who's wearing flip flops."
❋ Repeat until there is only one person remaining, who becomes caller for the next round.

PERFECT FOR PARTIES

FUN FOR THE WHOLE FAMILY

BIG GROUP FUN

INDOOR OR OUTDOOR:
Both

AGES:
5 and older

HOW MANY CAN PLAY?
At least 8,
but 12 is much better

WEATHER:
If outside, warm and dry

TIME REQUIRED:
At least 15 minutes

PARENTAL SUPERVISION/ INVOLVEMENT:
Need a responsible preteen or adult to remove chairs

INTENSITY LEVEL:
Easy

SAMPLE FRUIT BASKET STATEMENTS

Come up with your own, noninsulting statements to indicate which people must get up out of their chairs, or try these:

I'm grateful for . . .
People with brown hair
People wearing socks
People with earrings
People whose grandma is here today
People who like chocolate ice cream best
People with glasses or contacts
People who are wearing shoes you tie
People who are wearing a hair clip
People who drink coffee
People who are 7 years old
People who can roll their tongue (demonstrate)
and so forth

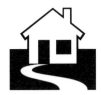

Blind Fetch

This is a dream game for a family holiday, all-adult picnic, or even a management retreat. Liken it to a verbal Pictionary form of tag... and like Pictionary, it's lots of fun for extended family bonding and includes a variety of age groups without being boring for older kids or adults.

What You Need

* Blindfolds (one for each team)
* Handball or small bouncy ball such as Spaldeen, a pink rubbery ball available at most toy stores or online.

Setting Up

* Divide the group into two or three teams of four or five each, and designate one person per team to wear the blindfold.
* Mark off the play area, an area of at least 15 feet by 15 feet, and mark lines on as many sides as you have teams.

How to Play

* Each team fans out along its designated side of the playing area, with all players standing behind the line.
* Once one player from each team is blindfolded, have one person (it doesn't matter who) toss the handball into the play area.

FUN FOR THE WHOLE FAMILY

BIG GROUP FUN

HOURS OF FUN

INDOOR OR OUTDOOR:
Both

AGES:
6 and older, and all adults is just fine

HOW MANY CAN PLAY?
2 to 18

WEATHER:
Moderate temperature, dry ground

TIME REQUIRED:
Starting with set-up, at least 30 minutes

PARENTAL SUPERVISION/ INVOLVEMENT:
Definitely makes it more fun, but not necessary after the blindfolds are on

INTENSITY LEVEL:
Easy to Moderate

✳ The blindfolded players then move into the playing area, following directions shouted to them by their teammates, who must stay behind the perimeter line of the playing area.

✳ Once a player finds the ball, he or she collects it. While still blindfolded, the player returns to his or her team based on instructions shouted from those teammates. If the player succeeds in crossing back over the line without being tagged by another blindfolded player, that team receives three points.

✳ If another team's blindfolded player tags her as she's heading back, that team receives one point.

✳ If a blindfolded player peeks, she's grounded until the next round and her team loses one point.

✳ After all but one player have been tagged, or the ball makes it back to one of the teams, whichever comes first, start another round, with another team member from each team trying to complete the same task.

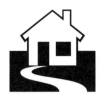

Sneaky Patty

This amusing exercise combines the best of Musical Chairs, Blindman's Bluff, and Tag, and still manages to be easy to understand for anyone who comprehends the basics of being sneaky.

WHAT YOU NEED

* Blindfold
* Chair
* CD player or boom box and music (or an old-fashioned record player)
* Teddy bear

SETTING UP

Stage the action where everyone can hear the music you'll play, preferably setting the chair in soft grass or on a carpet to muffle sounds and make it easier on the knees.

HOW TO PLAY

* Gather everyone into a circle and place a chair in the middle, then put the teddy bear under the chair.
* Blindfold the person who is It and seat him or her on the chair.
* Choose who will go first, and then turn on some music, playing it loud enough so that all players can hear it clearly.

* With the music disguising the sound of her movements, the first player will try to sneak up to the chair on his or her hands and knees and snatch the Teddy bear.

* The blindfolded child must stay seated, but can flail his or her hands, trying for a blind tag. If the seated child tags someone, that player has to switch places with him or her.

* After each child (working clockwise) has made one attempt, appoint another It if no one has been tagged.

* If people are getting tagged too easily, make the music a bit louder or restrict It to just one hand.

Birthday Party Fun. At a birthday party, consider putting the party favors under the chair instead, and each child can keep trying until he or she has retrieved a favor.

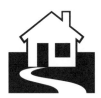

Hide and Seek

Hide and Seek is the stuff summer memories are made of. It doesn't matter whether the thrill of calling "ready or not" or sprinting for base are part of a family game, a sleepover, or just a big group of kids and parents at a park. The best part about Hide and Seek is that most people have at least a general idea of how to play. That's why it is so easy to organize with big groups. You can choose a variety that suits the area you have to play in—and one that assures enjoyment for the most players, the slow, the surly, and the sprinters all included.

WHAT YOU NEED

No equipment needed

SETTING UP

✳ Two to four backyards with plenty of hiding places are ideal for Hide and Seek, though it can also be played in a large house.

✳ Select an area of the playing field (tree, porch, lawn chair, and so on) as the "base."

NO EQUIPMENT NEEDED

FUN FOR THE WHOLE FAMILY

PERFECT FOR PARTIES

BIG GROUP FUN

INDOOR OR OUTDOOR:
Both

AGES:
7 and older

HOW MANY CAN PLAY?
6 or more

WEATHER:
If outside, warm and dry

TIME REQUIRED:
At least 15 minutes

PARENTAL SUPERVISION/ INVOLVEMENT:
Not necessary

INTENSITY LEVEL:
Easy to moderate

How to Play

✳ The person who is It stands by the designated base with eyes closed and counts to 100 by fives while the other players scramble to hide. If the playing field is very large, you should count to a greater number to allow enough time for the other players to hide.

✳ Once finished counting the person who is It yells, "Ready or not, here I come," and runs around trying to find the hiding players and tag them.

✳ Players must then try to get to the designated base without being tagged. The game proceeds in this way until all the players have either been tagged or have reached base.

Rules of Play

✳ The first player tagged becomes It for the next round of play.

✳ If no one has been tagged, the person who is It must keep that role for the next round.

✳ All players who make it to the base without being tagged are considered winners.

There are so many variations of Hide and Seek it would be nearly impossible to list them all, but these are tried and true.

MANHUNT

In this variation, when tagging a player you must hold on to them and repeat, "Manhunt, Manhunt, 1–2–3" three times; the player is not eliminated from the game if you can't hold on long enough to say this phrase. Players who have been tagged are disqualified from the game. The last person tagged becomes It for the next round of play.

HIDE AND RACE

If you are It in this version, you don't actually have to tag anyone. Instead, when you see a player, you yell, "One, two, three on (name the hiding player)." That player then races you to the base. If you get there first, he or she is out. If the player gets there first, he or she is safe. The first player who loses a race with you becomes It for the next game.

CHAIN HIDE AND SEEK

In this spin-off, players who are either tagged or spotted must join hands (or lock elbows) with It for the duration of the game. Play continues until all but one player have become part of the chain; this player is then It for the next round.

Indoor Balloon Race

Try this game as an active alternative to watching DVDs on a rainy afternoon—or at halftime when friends are over to watch a ballgame. There's no way to tell who has a natural ability to use a cardboard fan to propel a balloon forward, so anyone can win this game.

WHAT YOU NEED

* String
* Two balloons
* Two pieces of cardboard about the size of the side of a cereal box

SETTING UP

* In your backyard (or in a spacious room inside your house) mark two lines on the floor about 20 feet apart using a towel, toilet paper, or anything else that's handy.
* Divide players into two equal teams and have team members stand single file in two lines at the designated starting line.
* Each team gets a balloon with a string attached to the end, and a piece of cardboard.

How to Play

✳ Someone not playing the game yells, "On your marks. Get set. Go!" and the first player in each line throws the balloon up in the air.

✳ Players use the cardboard as a fan to keep the balloon airborne while they maneuver it to the 20-foot line, turn it around, and return to the starting line.

✳ While keeping the balloon airborne, the first player hands the cardboard over to the next player in line, who then repeats the process.

✳ The race continues in this way until all the members of one team have successfully maneuvered the balloon to the 20-foot line and back.

Rules of Play

✳ The balloon cannot touch the ground at any time.

✳ If a player loses control of the balloon and it touches the ground, he has to go back to the starting line and begin that leg of the race again.

✳ Only the cardboard can be used to fan the balloon. Players who blow on the balloon to maneuver it must start their leg of the race over again.

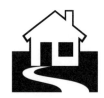

Limbo

If it's fun on a cruise ship, surely it will work for your group. This is a fun way to bend and shake and show some personality—and the younger, shorter, and more limber folks are at an advantage, which is really fun for them.

WHAT YOU NEED

✳ A broomstick or mop handle to use as a limbo bar.

SETTING UP

✳ Two players stand holding the limbo bar at about chest level.

HOW TO PLAY

✳ Players take turns trying to pass under the limbo bar without bending forward or touching the ground with their hands.
✳ The limbo bar is lowered to about waist level once all players have had a turn passing under it. Again, players take turns passing under the limbo bar at the reduced height.
✳ Play continues in this way, with the bar being lowered gradually and players taking turns trying to pass under it. The player who can go under the limbo bar at the lowest level is the winner.

FUN FOR THE WHOLE FAMILY

RAINY DAY FUN

BIG GROUP FUN

INDOOR OR OUTDOOR:
Both

AGES:
7 and older

HOW MANY CAN PLAY?
6 or more

WEATHER:
If outside, warm and dry

TIME REQUIRED:
At least 20 minutes

PARENTAL SUPERVISION/ INVOLVEMENT:
Not necessary, but fun

INTENSITY LEVEL:
Easy to Moderate

✳ Players are disqualified if they knock over the limbo bar, touch the ground with their hands, or fall down when going under the limbo bar.

WATER LIMBO

This cool version of Limbo is great on hot, steamy days when all you want to do is run through the sprinklers. All rules of play are the same, except instead of limbo-ing under the broomstick, your challenge is to pass under a stream of water. One player holds a garden hose at about chest level and makes the water jet out into a beam by putting a finger over half of the spout. The other players take turns trying to pass under the water jet without breaking the beam, falling down, or touching the ground with their hands. The water beam is lowered to about waist level when all players have had a chance to limbo. The game continues, with the beam being lowered a little bit after each round, until all but one player has been disqualified.

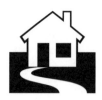

Conkers

This game is very English, and although it's not super active, it is super intriguing—you can spend hours perfecting your conker for maximum missile power, sort of like league bowlers pretreating their bowling balls—only cheaper. And you can play pretty much anywhere there's enough room for two people to stand and one of them to swing a conker. Start a trend with your friends and family and give away pre-strung conkers as inexpensive birthday gifts.

WHAT THE HECK IS A CONKER?

The smooth, small brown objects known as conkers are actually seeds of the horse chestnut. They are typically harvested in early autumn, but be wary as the brown chestnuts grow within super-spiny pods. It's best to find an open pod on the ground and pry the conker out by stepping on the opening with thick-soled athletic shoes. You might luck out and find one on the ground, too. If your neighborhood or park doesn't have a supply, hit up a street vendor who sells the roasted type, or try the gourmet market, but only buy the uncooked chestnuts that still have their brown skins on—not water chestnuts or peeled.

WHAT YOU NEED
* One conker for each player

HOURS OF FUN

INDOOR OR OUTDOOR:
Both, but indorrs in a gym or large room with no breakables

AGES:
8 and older—players need good hand-eye coordination

HOW MANY CAN PLAY?
2 or more

WEATHER:
Not raining or snowing and not too cold

TIME REQUIRED:
At least 25 minutes unless you've got a champ

PARENTAL SUPERVISION/ INVOLVEMENT:
An adult needs to drill a hole in each conker

INTENSITY LEVEL:
Easy, but takes lots of skill

SETTING UP

* Drill a hole though the conker so you can thread it an 18-inch piece of string through it. Tie a knot in the string so the conker won't come off.

HOW TO PLAY

* Decide who goes first by coin toss or by determining who has the most wins in her past record.
* In this scenario, the owner of a "fiver" (a conker that has won five of its previous games) has priority over the owner of a mere "two-er."
* The receiver holds out her hand at arm's length and dangles her conker on the end of its string, as if it were a fully-extended yo-yo.
* The other player then grasps the end of her conker string and attempts to swing her conker to hit the dangling conker as hard as she can. Overhanded swings are usually the rule.
* If the challenger makes solid contact with the dangling conker, she gets another go. If she misses, roles are reversed and the receiver gets a crack at her opponent.
* This continues until one or other of the conkers is so damaged that it falls off the string.

RULES OF PLAY

* You can decide whether play turns over if a conker hits a string instead of the other conker, or if underhanded swings are allowed.
* Once one of the conkers has been destroyed, the winner can add the loser's conker value to the victory count of his or her conker.

For example, if a fiver perservered over a two-er, the fiver would become a sevener.

STRATEGIES FOR MORE CAPABLE CONKING

There are lots of ways to treat a conker to make it stronger and more durable, but who knows if any of them work? No harm trying one (but only one—don't combine!) of the following

1. Soak your conker in vinegar for a week.
2. Bake the conker in a 250°F oven for 6 to 8 hours.
3. Cover your conker with a thin coat of clear nail polish.

Of course, your neighborhood Conker League might want to banish any or all of the above—or any other wacky technique a competitor can come up with.

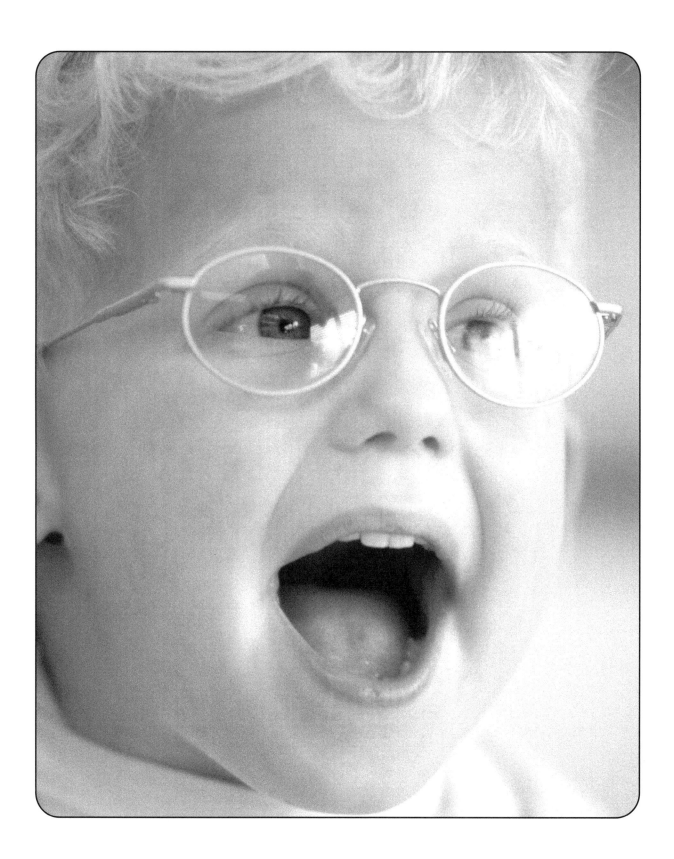

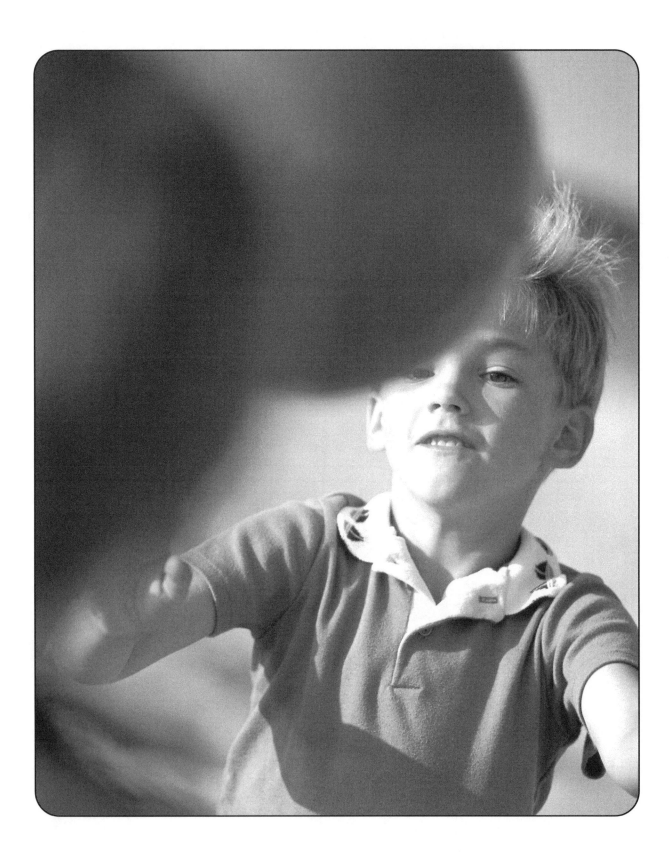

3

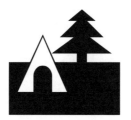

OUTDOOR GAMES

Even Donna Reed probably drew blank stares when she ordered the kids to "go out and get some fresh air, it's a beautiful day." Instead of telling, show kids how much fun playing outside can be with some organized— well, semi-organized—games. To avoid beginner's frustration, start small and simple with say, Follow the Leader or Simon Says, games that don't require much time or equipment. If you're planning an outdoor picnic or family reunion or even the activity for the soccer team party, take on something more ambitious, like Steal the Bacon or Kick the Can. Try to anticipate and prevent competitive whine fests by balancing teams and abilities—and varying the games to play to diverse strengths. Most important, view any combination of an empty space and a half-hour of downtime as an outdoor game possibility, from waiting on the museum steps to enjoying an evening from your suburban deck. And don't worry if the games don't go smoothly at first, or deteriorate into crazy running around—what's most important is to have fun and keep moving.

Dizzy Bat Race

This game is a popular distraction between innings at many minor league baseball games. It's an equally fun option for play groups, picnics, and family reunions. In fact, shorter kids have a bit of an advantage in this game, because they don't have to bend as far to get their foreheads on the bat, so it makes for a good mixed-age event, too.

WHAT YOU NEED

❋ One baseball bat for each player.

SETTING UP

Designate start and finish lines 10 feet to 30 feet apart (depending on how dizzy players are willing to get). Each player takes a baseball bat and stands at the starting line.

HOW TO PLAY

❋ Players put one end of the bat on the ground, bend over, and lean their foreheads on the other end of the bat.

❋ A person who isn't participating in the game calls out, "On your marks. Get set. Go!" And players run in a circle as quickly as possible while keeping their foreheads in contact with the bat.

INDOOR OR OUTDOOR:
Outdoor

AGES:
3 and older

HOW MANY CAN PLAY?
2 or more

WEATHER:
Warm and dry

TIME REQUIRED:
At least 15 minutes

PARENTAL SUPERVISION/ INVOLVEMENT:
Not necessary

INTENSITY LEVEL:
Easy

✳ After five turns, players drop their bats and run toward the finish line. The first player to cross the finish line and remain standing is the winner.

RULES OF PLAY

✳ If a player's forehead loses contact with the bat he must stop, reestablish contact, and continue counting turns from where he left off.

✳ To make the game more challenging you can increase the number of required turns, and the distance between the start and finish lines.

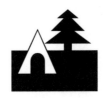

Pop Bottle Ring Toss

A favorite at elementary school fairs, this game is fun for the youngest, but can still lure older kids and adults who have decent hand-eye coordination. Play for prizes the first time, then let the kids set it up for the adults the next time around.

WHAT YOU NEED

* Two-liter soda bottles, at least eight of them.
* Plastic rings at least 10 inches in diameter (available at toy stores)—or make rings from paper plates by cutting a circle out of the middle of the plate and leaving the rim.

SETTING UP

* Fill empty soda bottles with sand or water. If you're feeling fancy, buy colored sand from the craft store and use that.
* Place the soda bottles in a diamond pattern on the basement floor, in the sand at the beach, or on a flat surface in the back yard, but far enough apart so that the rings can shimmy to the bottom if a player manages to toss a ring over a bottle.

HOW TO PLAY

❉ Players stand behind a line and try to toss the rings onto the bottles.

❉ Each player gets five rings, and the player who gets the most rings around the bottles wins.

VARIATIONS ON THE THEME

Increase the Challenge. Make the game more challenging by using different sizes of bottles, smaller rings, or by placing the bottles closer together.

Message on the Bottle. For a party, wrap small slips of paper around the neck of the bottle, each explaining what prize the one who loops that bottle will take home. For at-home family fun, make the messages a mix of privileges and chores, with each family member taking luck of the draw, mom and dad included.

Make It, Take It. For PTA fairs or beach gatherings, use unopened 20-ounce bottles. Make the rings smaller, more like five inches. You'll have to cut smaller holes on the paper plates, or use dessert-size plates. Then let players take whichever beverages they ring. You may want to limit winners to two sodas probably, unless you're taking a fee for entry!

The Great Pumpkin Toss. Place a good-size pumpkin 8 feet to 10 feet ahead of you on the ground, and practice tossing hula hoops over it, giving one point per score. Once this becomes too easy, move the pumpkin farther back.

Get Frosty. After you build that perfect snowman, back up eight paces and take turns trying to fling his hat onto his head. Award two points if the hat lands on top of his head, one if it is askew. Keep score with all the players using the one hat, or just build more snowmen and see who gets hats on the most.

Capture the Stump. To soothe the grief over losing a tree in the yard (and maybe the pain of having to pay for it to be cut down), try the hula-hoop ring toss with the stump (see Great Pumpkin Toss, above). Or you can practice throwing kernels of dry corn onto the stump for the birds and squirrels from just a few steps, not a few yards, away. It's a great way to work on aim and your underhand pitch, and boy can that corn bounce if you throw it too hard.

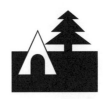

Red Light, Green Light

NO EQUIPMENT NEEDED

SUPER-QUICK

INDOOR OR OUTDOOR:
Outdoor

AGES:
5 and older

HOW MANY CAN PLAY?
4 or more

WEATHER:
Moderate temperatures, wind okay, not raining, but a little water on the ground okay

TIME REQUIRED:
Maybe 15 minutes

PARENTAL SUPERVISION/ INVOLVEMENT:
Not necessary

INTENSITY LEVEL:
Easy

Make sure to enjoy lots of rounds of this game with your children before they're all too soon taking the wheel of a real car and watching out for the real traffic lights. It's a great chance to run around and let off a little steam, and super fun for sneaky kids. Play anytime you need a 10-minute break and have a few yards of free earth—or even a driveway.

What You Need

No equipment needed.

Setting Up

* A large backyard is ideal for this game.
* One player is selected to be the Stoplight for the first round of play. She stands with her back to the other players.
* Players line up at a designated starting point about 10 yards away from the Stoplight. You can vary this distance depending on how long you want the game to last.

How to Play

* The Stoplight stands with her back to the other players and yells "Green Light." All players begin running toward her as fast as they can.

✳ The Stoplight then yells, "Red Light," and turns around quickly. All players must stop running immediately, and remain motionless. Any players seen moving by the Stoplight are disqualified.

TIP FOR THE STOPLIGHT

Try to confuse the runners by yelling "Red light" and "Green light" at varying time intervals. After you've called "Green light," wait three seconds and yell "Red light." Wait 30 seconds before calling "Green light," so the runners stop paying attention, and then quickly yell "Red Light" again.

STOPPING SHORT

If you're playing on grass and you hear the Stoplight yell "Red Light," you need to stop moving as soon as possible. When you're running fast it might be difficult to stop short without falling down—it might help to drop on your knees or roll on the ground. If you're playing on a hard surface, pay close attention to your speed so that you can stop without falling down and hurting yourself.

RULES OF PLAY

✳ When the Stoplight yells "Red Light," running players are given 2 seconds to come to a complete stop.

✳ The player who reaches the Stoplight first is the winner, and becomes the Stoplight in the next round of play.

✳ If all players are disqualified, the Stoplight is the winner, and remains the Stoplight for the next round of the game.

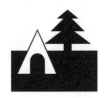

Five Dollars

It's baseball, sort of, but with no seventh-inning stretch nor catcher's masks and such required. If kids already know baseball basics, this will help them hone their batting and fielding skills. If baseball doesn't run in the family bloodlines, you'll pick up a bit of lingo (fly, grounder, outfield) and some basic concepts about batting—without committing to tedious hours of rules and learning positions. This is a nice game for softball-playing moms and dads to take time to play with the neighborhood horde.

What You Need

* Wiffle bat or Fun Gripper Bat.
* Wiffle ball or Fun Gripper Ball.

Setting Up

* If you live near a school or ballpark and you can use the field, you're all set. Otherwise, play in a field or backyard that is at least a half acre and not near breakable windows, expensive landscaping, or parked cars.
* Set up a "home plate" some 5 yards from one edge of the field.
* Send everyone else out to face the home plate.

How to Play

❋ The batter tosses the light ball into the air and then bats it to the outfield. Or, he uses a batting tee, or someone in the outfield tosses him a pitch, depending on the players' experience level and what will yield the most fly balls and solid hits.

❋ Outfielders try to catch the ball. They win points depending on how well and quickly they field the hits.

Rules of Play

❋ Outfielders receive points as follows: One dollar for each fly catch, 50 cents for a one-bounce catch, 25 cents for fielding a grounder (one that bounces more than once or rolls along the ground).

❋ The first person to receive 5 dollars bats next.

❋ To make the game a little easier on the wallet, award points instead of cash (three points for a fly catch, two points for a one-bounce catch, and one point for fielding a grounder). The first person to receive five points bats next.

Tips for Younger Kids

If no one can really bat the ball high enough or far enough to make the game fun, use a T-ball batting tee, available inexpensively at chain toy or sporting goods stores. Or, have only a single batter, one who's more experienced, and let the little kids field. P.S.: The kids won't even realize that they are practicing math!

Tips for the Outfielder

Try to position yourself in a spot away from the others, up closer if possible, or "out in left field." That way, you won't have to fight for every ball, but should catch something every now and then. This is also a good spot for a less-skilled player. Finally, remind the batter to lob a few easy ones.

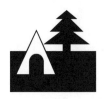

Cat and Mouse

Forget what you've seen when your house cat has its unblinking eye on real or imagined prey. This game is fun and active, and takes almost no patience at all. You will be learning the basic concepts of teamwork, though, and also start getting used to the idea of calling out perfectly ridiculous statements in the time-honored tradition of family games.

WHAT YOU NEED

No equipment needed

SETTING UP

One player is selected to be the Cat, and another to be the Mouse.

HOW TO PLAY

✳ Players form a circle and hold hands.
✳ The Cat waits outside the circle until the Mouse enters the circle and yells, "I am the Mouse! You can't catch me!" The Cat responds, "I am the Cat! We'll see, we'll see!"
✳ The Cat tries to enter the circle to catch the Mouse while players try to keep him out.

NO EQUIPMENT NEEDED

PERFECT FOR PARTIES

BIG GROUP FUN

SUPER-QUICK

INDOOR OR OUTDOOR:
Outdoors

AGES:
5 and older

HOW MANY CAN PLAY?
6 or more

WEATHER:
Warm and dry

TIME REQUIRED:
At least 10 minutes

PARENTAL SUPERVISION/ INVOLVEMENT:
Not necessary

INTENSITY LEVEL:
Easy to moderately active

Rules of Play

* Players keep their hands joined and move close together to keep the Cat outside of the circle.

* Players drop their hands to let the mouse out of the circle if the Cat gets in.

* The Mouse becomes part of the circle when he gets caught, and a new Cat is chosen for the next round of play.

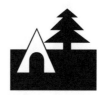

Mother May I

Mother May I is so fun and silly your kids won't even notice they're getting a bit of exercise. No wonder it's always been a school-yard favorite. You can play a speedy game or leave off and pick it up another time, too, so be sure to work in a quick game at the bus stop, for example, or with the group of kids who are waiting for sister to finish ballet lessons. Remember any favorite steps from your earlier playing days? If not, make up whatever you can and always remember to throw in a few "backward" for good effect.

What You Need

No equipment needed

Setting Up

* A large backyard is ideal for this game, or a driveway that's reasonably clear. Play it in the park, too.
* One player is selected to be Mother for the first round of play. All other players should stand in a row about 20 feet to 30 feet away from Mother.

How to Play

* Mother calls the name of a player and tells her to take a certain number of steps.
* When giving instructions Mother also specifies the kind of step (baby, giant, hop, and so on) and in what

NO EQUIPMENT NEEDED

PERFECT FOR PARTIES

INDOOR OR OUTDOOR:
Outdoor

AGES:
5 and up

HOW MANY CAN PLAY?
3 or more

WEATHER:
Warm and dry

TIME REQUIRED:
At least 15 minutes

PARENTAL SUPERVISION/ INVOLVEMENT:
Not necessary

INTENSITY LEVEL:
Easy

direction (forward, backward, left, or right) to take it. For example, Mother calls out "Jack, you may take one baby step forward."

✳ Jack should then ask, "Mother, may I?" to which Mother can respond "Yes you may," "No you may not," or even "No you may not. Instead take two hopping steps backward."

RULES OF PLAY

✳ If players don't respond to Mother's instructions with "Mother, may I," they must return to the starting line and begin again.

✳ The first player to cross the imaginary line where Mother is standing is the winner, and becomes Mother for the next round of play.

TIPS FOR MOTHER

When it's your turn to be Mother, try to be creative with your instructions. Vary the number and type of steps you give, as well as the directions. Tell the players to hop, skip, walk like a chicken, or even roll on the ground. Use your imagination—no movement is too silly.

STEP IDEAS

Hop on one foot
Baby step (backward)
Chug like a train
Flap your arms like a chicken
Gallop
Giant step (backward)
Hobble with a "cane"
Hop like a kangaroo
Jump backward
Leap like a frog

Skip
Tip toe
Twirl like a ballerina
Umbrella step (spinning, arms extended to form an "umbrella" from your shoulders)
Walk with your hands behind your head
Zoom like a plane

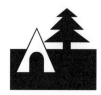

Queenie

This game is part bluff, part hustle, and you can play it almost anywhere—a backyard, driveway, school playground, in a pool, or on the beach. It's a subtle chance to work on your child's fielding and hand-eye coordination, too. Just don't let the neighborhood "fetching" dog get wind that you're starting a game.

WHAT YOU NEED

* A fist-size ball with some bounce such as a tennis ball or a pink rubbery Spaldeen, available at most toy stores.

SETTING UP

Players form a loose circle. Queenie stands 10 feet to 15 feet away holding the ball.

HOW TO PLAY

* One player is chosen to be Queenie.
* Queenie turns around, so she can't see the other players, and throws the ball over her head toward the circle.
* Players scramble to get the ball. When it has been caught, players re-form the circle and stand with their hands behind their backs. Once everyone is in position, the group yells, "Ready."

PERFECT FOR PARTIES

SUPER-QUICK

INDOOR OR OUTDOOR:
Outdoor

AGES:
5 and older

HOW MANY CAN PLAY?
4 or more

WEATHER:
Warm and dry

TIME REQUIRED:
5 minutes per round, tops

PARENTAL SUPERVISION/ INVOLVEMENT:
Not necessary

INTENSITY LEVEL:
Easy

✴ Queenie then turns to face the group and guesses which player is hiding the ball.

TIPS FOR FOOLING QUEENIE

Work as a team to keep Queenie from guessing correctly. When Queenie turns around, several players should try to look nervous or guilty to make it seem like they have the ball. Other players can wink at each other, or make secret gestures to confuse Queenie even more.

RULES OF PLAY

✴ Queenie gets only one chance to identify the player with the ball.
✴ If she guesses correctly, she stays Queenie for the next round of play; if she chooses incorrectly, then the person hiding the ball becomes Queenie.

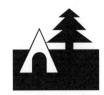

Wheelbarrow Race

If you are organized enough to host a family field day, this should be a staple event. It's active and rewards strength and coordination, but even when you don't succeed, you get lots of hilarity and laughter. Best of all, this game is easiest for light, nimble little kids who love to best the grown-ups every now and then.

What You Need

No equipment needed

Setting Up

Using markers such as garden hoses or towels, designate a starting line and a finishing line 15 feet to 30 feet apart.

How to Play

❋ At the starting line, one person from each pair gets down on her hands and knees and lifts her feet off the ground so her partner can pick up her ankles.

❋ When the race starts, the partner on the ground begins "running" on her hands while her partner holds up her ankles.

❋ The first team to cross the finish line wins the race.

NO EQUIPMENT NEEDED

FUN FOR THE WHOLE FAMILY

PERFECT FOR PARTIES

BIG GROUP FUN

INDOOR OR OUTDOOR:
Outdoor

AGES:
5 and older

HOW MANY CAN PLAY?
2 or more teams of 2

WEATHER:
Warm and dry

TIME REQUIRED:
At least 20 minutes

PARENTAL SUPERVISION/ INVOLVEMENT:
Not necessary

INTENSITY LEVEL:
Easy

TIPS FOR TEAMMATES: DON'T PUSH TOO FAST

When you are the standing partner be careful not to push your teammate forward too quickly or too hard. Remember that it's a lot harder to "run" with all your weight on your hands, and nobody wants to land face first in the grass.

RULES OF PLAY

The partner on the ground must keep his or her knees raised throughout the race—if they touch the ground at any time, the team must return to the starting line and begin the race again.

WHEELBARROW SWITCH RACE

For this variation, find a favorite cousin or grab a willing sibling to team up for hands-on fun. Just as in a classic wheelbarrow race, one player is the wheelbarrow and "walks" on her hands. Her partner holds her feet and "pushes" the wheelbarrow as they careen to the finish. In this version, partners race to a line, switch positions, and race back.

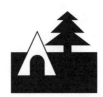

Basic Relay

In any relay, teams move back and forth along some sort of course to finish tasks and win a race against other teams. These tasks can be a serious aerobic workout, a distance jog or short sprint—or just some preposterous gimmicks to promote fun and foolishness. Choose sides, mark off a distance, both a start and a finish line, and then pick your fun with any variation you choose.

What You Need

Varies depending upon which relay game you play (see below).

Setting Up

Varies depending upon which relay game you play (see below).

How to Play

Varies depending upon which relay game you play (see below).

Rules of Play

The basic rules of play are the same for every relay variation:

❋ No member of a relay team can run (or perform any other task) twice before the whole team has participated once.

❋ When team members pass an object—whether it's an egg in a spoon or a soccer ball—the pass must occur behind the starting line to qualify.

PERFECT FOR PARTIES

BIG GROUP FUN

INDOOR OR OUTDOOR:
Outdoor

AGES:
6 and up

HOW MANY CAN PLAY?
6 or more, at least 10 preferred

WEATHER:
If outdoors, warm and dry

TIME REQUIRED:
At least 15 minutes

PARENTAL SUPERVISION/ INVOLVEMENT:
Parents should play and organize

INTENSITY LEVEL:
Easy to moderate

A Roundup of Relay Variations

BUCKET BRIGADE

Each team places an empty bucket at the finish line, and a bucket full of water at the start line, which is 20 feet away from the finish line. The teams line up, single file, at the start line so that each team has a first "runner" who stands next to that team's bucket of water. This first runner holds a cup. On "Go!" each runner dips water into the cup and races to the finish line to pour it into the empty bucket. Each runner then returns to pass his or her cup to the next runner on the team. The first team to fill their bucket (to the top or past a certain marked line) wins.

LEAKY CUP

Instead of a measuring cup, give each team a large paper or Styrofoam cup, in the bottom of which you have made a small pin hole. Runners dip the cup into the water bucket and then put it on their head while they run—no hands. All the other rules are the same.

HULA HOOP

Each person must walk the course while they keep a Hula Hoop in motion around their hips. Better make this course just about 5 feet to begin with—this variation is harder than it sounds.

Apple Roll

Each team must roll an apple across the grass with a Popsicle stick, on a course that's about 5 feet long. After crossing the finish line, the runner then runs back to the starting line to pass the apple and stick to the next contestant. The pass must occur behind the starting line.

Keep 'Em Kicking Relay

This version is perfect for budding soccer players or for some really active kids who need to burn off energy at a picnic. Have each player dribble (kick in short distances) a soccer ball to a marker some 20 yards away and back. No fair kicking farther than a yard at the time. Any player who does has to start over.

MORE KICKING RELAYS

Add an element of balance to any kicking relay by having players carry an egg in a spoon as they dribble the ball through the course. Touching the egg or the bowl of the spoon is forbidden. For this you may wish to shorten the course to 10 yards or less.

Change the game again by telling players they may kick only with their "off" foot. Players who favor their right foot must use the left only, and vice versa.

Tell players they must put the ball on the ground when they reach the halfway marker and jog around it three times before coming back.

If you have a mixture of super-athletic and less athletic players, you can even out the competition by having them stop at the marker to sing three verses of the Farmer in the Dell.

Chin-to-Chin Pass

Look, Ma, no hands! Revisit hip cocktail party games from the sixties and pass with your chin. Standing side by side, each team in one line, pass a piece of fruit, a tennis ball or even a water balloon from chin to chin, down the line to the last player. (Reaching the last player is the object, not covering the distance). The first team to pass the object without dropping it wins. If a team member does drop the object, that team must start again at the beginning of the line. Or, for a less harsh variation, re-start with the same player who dropped it.

CRAYON CRAZINESS

Each team receives one box of 16 crayons. Give one or two crayons to each runner, and place the empty boxes at a finish line at least 10 yards away. Teams race to fill the crayon boxes, crayon by crayon. Choose your "anchor," or last, runner carefully, since the box has to be able to be closed completely before you declare a winner.

ONE SHOE OFF

Gather a shoe from everybody and pile them all up at a line some 15 yards from the starting line. The goal? Each person in the relay runs to pile with just one shoe, sorts her shoe out from the others, puts it on and runs to tag hands with the next runner on her team. Tip: Put the youngest (or slowest) player on the end of the relay, so she'll have fewer shoes to sort through.

WET HEAD RELAY

You must have nerves of steel and players who are good sports for this one. Each team designates one person to lie on her back across the halfway line, with an open, empty sports drink bottle on her forehead. The other players on the relay run, one at a time, from the starting point 20 yards away, carrying a paper cup of water (filled with drinkable water). At the halfway marker, the relay member attempts to fill the sports drink bottle with the water, which is still sitting on the teammate's forehead). Then the player runs back to tag the next player, and hand over the paper cup to fill with water. The winner is the team that fills the bottle first. Very strict rule: The player laying down may not use her hands to steady the bottle.

Balloon Relay

This is a race for relays made up of pairs, so each team should have an even number of players. Each relay member should choose a partner. Set a starting line and halfway point about 10 yards from each other, and give each team an inflated (not helium) balloon. On "Go!," the first two players in each relay run to the turning point. The trick is that the two players must keep a balloon in the air, batting it back and forth as they run to the finish. You can play with no hands for additional challenge.

Dress-Up Relay

Undress for success in this relay, and have a camera ready. You'll need it. Give each team a cardboard of oversize old clothes—and we don't mean coordinated outfits. A good combination is a big T-shirt, oversize shorts or skirt (if the boys and men all agree), fuzzy slippers, a man's jacket or blazer, an apron, and a hat and scarf. The first player puts on the clothing items (over his or her own clothes) and runs to a marker some 10 yards away and back. At the starting line, the next teammate helps the first teammate undress in order to put on the crazy outfit herself. To win, all players on a team must complete the course with all the clothes on—and the last player must remove the clothes and put them back in the box.

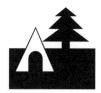

Capture the Flag

Capture the Flag can really get your hearts beating with exertion and anticipation. It's a super group game, because it draws equally from the strengths of the athletically gifted, the daring, and the tactician. Try to pick teams that have a fair smattering of each, and make sure an adult plays the first couple times until some adolescent-leadership emerges. It's a good way for kids to play out good-natured rivalries, but if there are real issues, put rivals on the same squad to avoid a bitter feud.

What You Need

❄ Two flags, or two objects that serve as flags—a shirt, rag, or jacket are all suitable.

Setting Up

❄ The ideal playing field ranges over three or four backyards, though a smaller terrain can be used.

❄ A "prison" area is designated on each side of the playing field.

❄ The playing field is divided into two equal halves, one for each team.

❄ Players on each side work together to hide the flag somewhere in their team's territory.

❄ Once the flags are hidden, each side signals the other that they're ready to begin.

BIG GROUP FUN

INDOOR OR OUTDOOR:
Outdoor

AGES:
7 and up

HOW MANY CAN PLAY?
2 teams of 3 or more

WEATHER:
Warm and dry

TIME REQUIRED:
At least 15 minutes for each round

PARENTAL SUPERVISION/ INVOLVEMENT:
Not necessary

INTENSITY LEVEL:
Active

How to Play

※ Players try to find the opposing team's flag and bring it back to their side of the field without being tagged. Players who have been tagged must wait in the opposing team's prison area for a member of their own team to come "free" them. The game ends when one team catches the opponent's flag.

Rules of Play

※ Players can only be tagged when on the opposing team's side of the playing field.

※ To be released from the prison area players must be tagged by one of their team members.

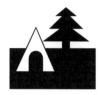

Steal the Bacon

Here's a game for those who like plays on words and physically active games. You can mesmerize those under age 8 or so if an adult will agree to be caller for a few rounds. Caller is also a fun spot for a smart-alecky teenager. This is the stuff suburban summer nights and city-park family picnics are made of. Once you learn all the rules, play often—Steal the Bacon is a game of strategy, loyalty, and subtle nuance that gets more fun the more people know what they're doing.

NUMBERS MATTER

You can tag only the opponent who shares the same number as you, so make sure to pay attention at the beginning of the game when the numbers are assigned, especially if you're playing with large teams.

WHAT YOU NEED

❋ A beanbag, tennis ball, can, or something similar to use as the "bacon"

SETTING UP

The ideal playing field is a large grassy backyard with at least 40 feet of open space.

❋ Using a rope, or anything else that's handy, mark two "home" lines (one for each team) 20 feet to 60 feet

BIG GROUP FUN

INDOOR OR OUTDOOR:
Outdoor

AGES:
7 and up

HOW MANY CAN PLAY?
7 or more

WEATHER:
Warm and dry

TIME REQUIRED:
At least 20 minutes

PARENTAL SUPERVISION/ INVOLVEMENT:
Not necessary, but fun

INTENSITY LEVEL:
Easy

apart, and then mark a third line to indicate the midline of the playing field.

✳ Select one player as the Caller. Divide all other players else into two equal teams and assign matching numbers (each team will have a "one," "two," and so on).

The Caller places the "bacon" on the midline of the playing field and then each team lines up at their designated home line.

How to Play

✳ The caller yells a number, and the players with that number on each team run toward the midline and try to grab the bacon.

✳ Once a player has the bacon he must return it to his team's home line before being tagged by his opponent.

✳ When players have reached their home lines the Caller returns the bacon to the midline, and yells another number.

✳ Play continues in this way until a predetermined number of points are scored, or until all numbers have been called.

Rules of Play

✳ Players can't tag each other until the bacon has been touched. For example, once their number has been called, players from each team can hover over the midline and tease each other while waiting for an opportunity to "steal the bacon." As long as neither has touched the bacon, no tagging can begin.

✳ Players score points by either bringing the bacon to their team's home line without being tagged, or by tagging their opponent before he carries the bacon to his team's home line.

✳ The Caller can yell out more than one number at a time. In this case, players from both teams whose numbers were called all run to the center and try to steal the bacon. Once the bacon has been touched, a player can only tag the opponent who shares the same number as him (number 5 can only tag number 5; number 2 can't tag number 1).

❋ If the caller yells "bacon" all players from both teams are allowed to rush to the midline for a chance to try to steal the bacon.

FUN FOR THE CALLER

Just because you're not running around with the other players doesn't mean you can't have just as much fun. When it's your turn to be the Caller make up word games when you yell out numbers; you'll confuse players who are paying attention and surprise those who aren't. Here are a few ideas to get you started.

"I drank six glasses of water today." Number 6 players run to steal the bacon.

"What are you two waiting for?" Players 2 and 4 on both teams rush for the midline.

"Did anyone have bacon for breakfast this morning?" All players on both teams head toward the midline to steal the bacon.

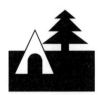

Dodgeball

● ●

BIG GROUP FUN

INDOOR OR OUTDOOR:
Outdoor

AGES:
7 and older

HOW MANY CAN PLAY?
2 teams of 6 or more

WEATHER:
Warm and dry

TIME REQUIRED:
At least 15 minutes

PARENTAL SUPERVISION/ INVOLVEMENT:
Yes, an adult needs to make sure the game doesn't go from intense to violent

INTENSITY LEVEL:
Moderate to Very Active

Playing Dodgeball is the ultimate way to increase your heart rate. You can't help but move around, or you'll get beaned! Beware of the potential for bullying or hard throws, though, and opt for a very soft ball if you have kids (or adults, for that matter) who might start taking the competition too seriously.

What You Need

✳ The number of balls to use depends on the number of players on each team, and on the desired pace of the game—four balls among eight players would make for a faster, more intense game than four balls between 16 players.

✳ Garden hose, jump rope, or other divider to break the playing field into two equal parts.

Setting Up

A large backyard, ideally with a fenced in area, is best suited for Dodgeball. Lay out the marker to divide the field into two playing areas.

How to Play

✳ Set the balls along the divider.

✳ At a pre-arranged "Go!" signal, players from both teams race to be the first to collect the balls.

✳ Those with the balls then throw them across the divider at the other team's players, trying to eliminate them from the game by hitting them below the waist.

RULES OF PLAY

✳ Team members must stay on their side of the field at all times.
✳ Players can deflect a thrown ball with a ball in their hands and still remain in the game.
✳ Players hit below the waist are disqualified. If a player is hit above the waist the player who threw the ball is out of the game.
✳ If a player catches a ball in the air (before it hits the ground) the player who threw it is disqualified.
✳ Players who try to catch a ball that is below waist level and drop it are disqualified.
✳ Any part of your body that is below waist level is fair game. For example, players who crouch down to catch the ball and get hit at a point relative to below waist level are disqualified. If the point of contact is comparably higher than waist level the player is still in, and the thrower is disqualified.

Any number of balls (one to six) can be used in each of the following dodgeball variations—it all depends on how quick or intense you want the game to be.

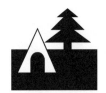

Dodgeball Variations for Ages 5 and Older

BUTT BALL

This is a great variation for younger children that can be played in backyards or spacious, uncluttered basements. In both cases, players are split into two teams and the playing area divided in half. The rules are the same as for regular Dodgeball with the exception of one: A player who deflects the ball with her butt is not eliminated from play. If a player is hit anywhere else below the waist, she is out. For example, if the ball is coming at a player she can dodge it completely, or turn around quickly and position her body so that her butt deflects the ball. Be considerate and don't throw the ball too hard—remember, butts are sensitive, too!

Tips for Indoor Play. Use softer balls than you would outside to avoid damaging your home or furniture, or hurting each other. Try any foam or Nerf balls, or even stuffed keepsake soccer balls.

INDOOR NERF BALL

For this indoor version of the game a soft ball (like Nerf) is needed. The playing area should be an uncluttered open space where you won't worry too much about breaking anything. The object of the game is to keep the ball moving without dropping it. Players stand in a circle and quickly throw the ball to each other. Anyone who drops the ball sits down on the floor, and the standing players continue with the game. The last standing player is the winner.

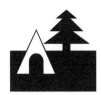

Dodgeball Variations for Ages 7 and Older

Older kids are faster and can handle more complex strategies and rules. Still use one to six balls, though, using more if you want the game to go faster and provide more of a workout.

CIRCLE DODGEBALL

Although players are divided into two equal teams for this spin-off, a single player will be the winner. One team forms a circle and the players on the other team spread out inside the circle. Players in the outer circle throw balls at the players inside; when a player is hit below the waist he is out. Play continues in this way until only one player is left inside the circle, and then teams switch positions—the team that was throwing now has to dodge.

CROSSOVER DODGEBALL

The object of this variation is to get all the players on one side of the playing field. After a player is hit, he crosses over the divider line and continues playing as a member of the opposing team.

FOUR-COURT DODGEBALL

After you have divided the playing field into two equal parts, and separated the players into two equal teams, designate a "bunker" behind the field on each team's side and mark it with another divider. One player from each team begins the game in the bunker on the opponent's side. He can throw balls to try to get the opposing team out—but only if someone from his own team can supply him with a ball or he manages to catch a stray shot, since he must remain within the bunker at all times. When a player is hit below the waist he goes to the bunker on the opponent's side and must remain inside to continue the game from there. When all the players of one team are in the bunker, the opposing team is declared the winner.

DOCTOR AND SPY

This unique version of Dodgeball can go on forever if both sides are crafty enough. Each team forms a huddle and chooses one player to be the Doctor and one to be the Spy. The Doctor can touch eliminated players to bring them back into the game. At any time during the game the facilitator (this can be any person not playing) can yell "Spy! 10 seconds!" Once this phrase is called, the designated Spy on each team can take a ball over to the opposing team's side of the playing field and try to hit and eliminate players for 10 seconds. The Spy must be back on his side of the playing field by the time the facilitator counts to 10 or he is out. Game play continues (following standard rules) until all the players of one team have been eliminated.

CAN YOU KEEP A SECRET?

The identity of the Doctor and the Spy should be kept secret from the opposing team for as long as possible. Once their identities are discovered, your opponents will try to eliminate them as soon as possible. When it's your turn to be the Doctor, be discreet when you tag eliminated players. Try bumping into your teammate "accidentally" or falling down near them and tagging a foot. Eliminated players can also help trick the other team by not returning to the game immediately after being tagged by the Doctor—this is a great way to keep the Doctor's identity a secret.

TEAMWORK PAYS OFF

The Doctor and the Spy are both valuable assets to your team—so work together as a group to protect them from being hit. The longer the Doctor remains in the game the more eliminated players he can bring back in to play. And don't forget about the Spy—if you lose him early in the game your team will be at a great disadvantage when the facilitator calls out, "Spy! 10 seconds!"

FRISBEE DODGE

You'll need a few (two to four) Frisbees for this fast-paced Dodgeball spin-off. Divide the playing field into two equal parts, and separate players into two equal teams. The object of the game is to eliminate players of the opposing team by hitting them with a Frisbee. As in many variations, if a player catches a Frisbee the player who threw it is out. Play continues until all players on one team are eliminated.

WALL BALL

There are no teams in this version of the game, so it's every man for himself. You'll need a big rubber ball and a long wall or the side of a house with no windows. Players line up in a loose row and the person who is It throws the ball against the wall and tries to hit another player below the waist on the bounce back. The player hit by the ball then becomes It for the next round of play. If a player gets hit above the waist, the thrower loses his turn as It, and a new It is chosen.

IT'S NOT JUST ABOUT BEING STRONG

In Wall Ball, accuracy and the ability to anticipate other players' moves are more important than just throwing the ball as hard as possible.

A DAVID AND GOLIATH TWIST

Prior to each round of play, each team picks a Goliath, and tells only the referees who it is. If the other team eliminates this Goliath, whether she's hit or throws a ball the other team catches, the whole team goes down. This makes the rounds end more quickly, and makes the brain work along with the body.

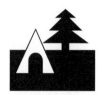

Ten Again

INDOOR OR OUTDOOR:
Outdoor

AGES:
7 and older

HOW MANY CAN PLAY?
5 or more

WEATHER:
Warm and dry

TIME REQUIRED:
At least 30 minutes

PARENTAL SUPERVISION/ INVOLVEMENT:
Not necessary

INTENSITY LEVEL:
Moderately to Very Active

This is the foot finesse version of Dodgeball. It's perfect for the kids who haven't developed throwing skills yet, and can also be a rigorous drill for your budding soccer star. Get an adult involved to keep the pace up—and to keep the bullying to a minimum.

What You Need

❋ Soccer ball (make it an indoor model) or a spongy, rubbery "playground ball" like the ones sold at any toy store. Also try a Fun Gripper Soccer Ball, available at toy stores or online.

Setting Up

❋ Designate one player to be It.
❋ Players form a large circle and the person who is It stands in the center.

How to Play

❋ Players get 10 chances to kick the ball at the person who is It.

Rules of Play

If the person who is It gets hit by the ball the player who kicked the ball becomes It for the next round of play. If the person who is It successfully dodges all 10 kicks he or she remains in the middle for one more round.

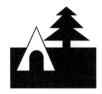

Red Rover

This perennial favorite from gym class is a great group game for the park or the yard after a family dinner. Be sure to put a leader on each team who is savvy and sympathetic and who can protect the younger and lesser skilled and make sure no one gets too vicious.

What You Need

No equipment needed.

Setting Up

Players are divided into two equal teams and stand 15 feet to 50 feet apart, depending on the desired intensity of the game. The closer the two teams, the milder the game and the more appropriate for younger players. The further apart you are, the more velocity a rowdy tackler can work up as he runs to toward the other line. Players on each team form a line, join hands, and face the opposing team.

How to Play

✽ Players from one team hold hands and yell, "Red Rover, Red Rover, send (an opposing player's name) right over!"

✽ The player whose name was called runs and tries to break through the line formed by his opponents (who are all holding hands).

NO EQUIPMENT NEEDED

PERFECT FOR PARTIES

BIG GROUP FUN

INDOOR OR OUTDOOR:
Outdoor

AGES:
7 and older

HOW MANY CAN PLAY?
2 teams of 4 or more players

WEATHER:
Warm and dry

TIME REQUIRED:
At least 15 minutes

PARENTAL SUPERVISION/ INVOLVEMENT:
A good idea, to keep it from getting vicious

INTENSITY LEVEL:
Moderately Active

✳ If the player breaks through the line, he chooses an opponent to take back to his team. If he doesn't break through, he joins the line of the opposing team.

✳ The game continues in this way, with teams taking turns calling out the Red Rover phrase.

✳ The game is over when only one player is left on a team.

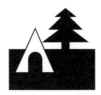

Share-A-Pair Race

This is sort of like a three-legged race, but with more, um, togetherness—and hence more laughs and fun. Groups of mixed ages will still have a great time, because the teams who do the best tend to be made up of same-size pairs, rather than the biggest players.

What You Need
❋ A pair of pantyhose or sweatpants for each pair of players—make sure the toes of the pantyhose have been cut off.

Setting Up
❋ Mark off a starting line that can accommodate how ever many pairs you have, and a finish line 40 yards to 50 yards away.
❋ Give each team their pair of pantyhose or sweatpants.

How to Play
❋ Each partner puts one leg into a leg of the hose or sweatpants that the team is sharing.
❋ On "Go!" each team member puts an arm around the other's shoulders and together they race to the finish line.

Rules of Play
❋ Both partners must cross the finish line with both feet still in the pants or hose and their arms around each others' shoulders to win.
❋ If a player's leg comes out of the sweatpants or pantyhose, she must return to that point to put the pants back on before starting to run again.

PERFECT FOR PARTIES

INDOOR OR OUTDOOR:
Outdoor

AGES:
7 and older

HOW MANY CAN PLAY?
even numbers 4 to 20

WEATHER:
Warm and dry

TIME REQUIRED:
At least 15 minutes

PARENTAL SUPERVISION/ INVOLVEMENT:
Yes

INTENSITY LEVEL:
Moderately to Very Active

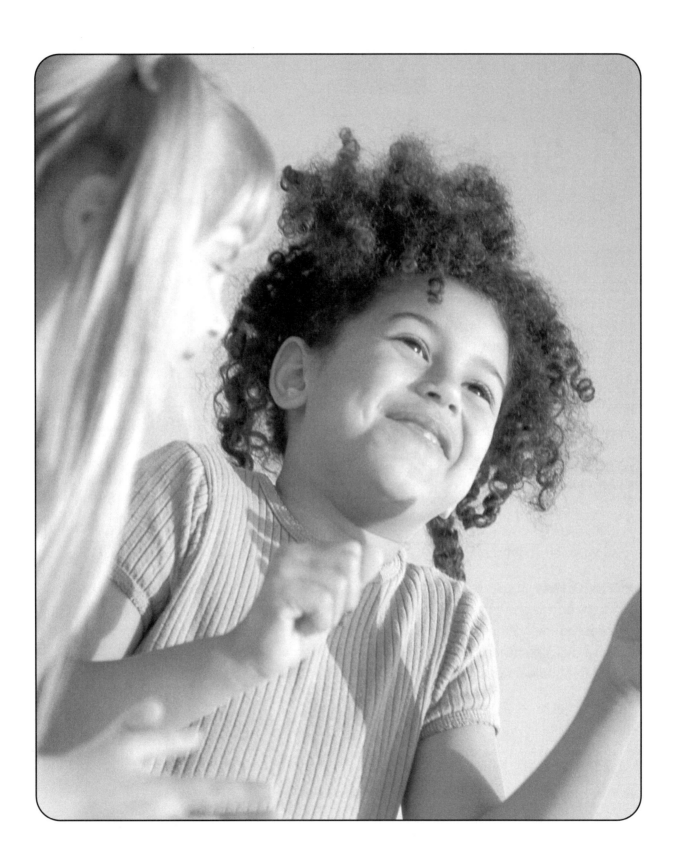

4

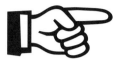

OUTDOOR TAG

Tag, You're It

HOW CAN I TAG YOU? LET ME COUNT THE WAYS...

You know the basic rules of tag already: One person is "It" and everyone else gets chased until one person is tagged. The first person tagged is the next It. Unfortunately, this plain-vanilla form of tag can devolve into a teasing session, with the slowest kids always being It. For the standard rules and then some new, improved models of the game, check out the following.

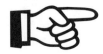

Basic Tag

Whether they are chasing kids on the playground or running after their siblings to get back a toy, children pretty much start playing tag when they learn to walk and keep at it... if they're active. You can encourage this physical activity and get moving yourself with a rousing game of standard tag. Once it has become a habit, you may choose to try some of the variations.

Be sure to remember tag as an option when you have a few free minutes in a place you can roam safely—like the rest stop on a long trip, or the square in front of the public library.

WHAT YOU NEED

No equipment needed.

SETTING UP

Choose a spot within the playing field (such as a specific tree, a porch, or a lawn chair) as the "base." Alternatively, any material (such as wood, metal, or concrete) can be designated as the base.

HOW TO PLAY

❋ All players except the person who is It start the game by touching the selected base. The person who is It counts to 100 by fives, and then yells, "Apples, peaches, pumpkin pie, anybody round my base is It!"

NO EQUIPMENT NEEDED

INDOOR OR OUTDOOR:
Outdoor

AGES:
5 and older (younger kids on adult shoulders)

HOW MANY CAN PLAY?
3 or more

WEATHER:
Moderate temperatures, and not too soggy

TIME REQUIRED:
At least 15 minutes

PARENTAL SUPERVISION/ INVOLVEMENT:
Not necessary, but fun

INTENSITY LEVEL:
Moderate to intense

✳ The person who is It chases the other players and tries to touch—or "tag"—them. When a player is touching the base, he is "safe" from It and cannot be tagged.

✳ When the person who is It catches another player he says, "Tag, you're It!" The tagged player then becomes It.

RULES OF PLAY

✳ A player cannot be tagged while he or she is touching the selected base, but only one person can touch base at a time, and he must move off after a count of 100.

✳ After the person who is It tags a player, he or she can avoid being immediately tagged back by saying, "You're It, no returns!" The player is then exempt from being tagged until after he or she returns to the base.

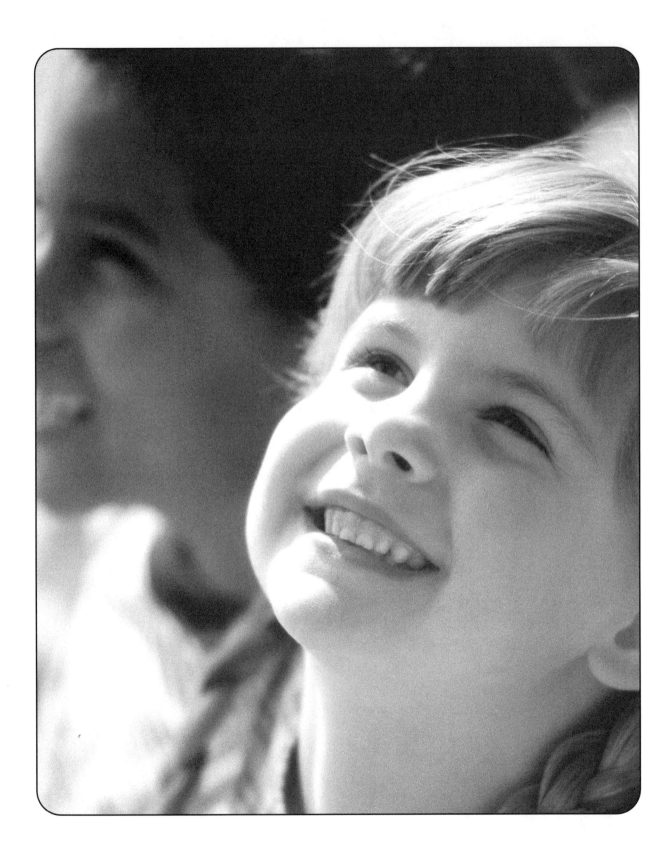

Tag Variations for Kids Ages 5 and Older

BODY TAG

In this spin-off, one player is designated It and another is chosen to be the "Judge." The rules are the same as in basic tag, except players are disqualified only if It tags the body part chosen by the Judge at the beginning of the round. For example, if the Judge calls "knees," players are out only if they get tagged on a knee. To stay in the game, players can run away from the person trying to tag them or simply shield the chosen body part from being tagged.

TIPS FOR THE JUDGE

When it's your turn to be the Judge, keep the other players on their toes by calling out a different body part every few minutes. Call out "shoulders," wait a while and then yell, "feet." Also, don't forget about smaller body parts. Pinky toes, noses, and ears are all fair game.

TAKE BODY TAG TO THE POOL

Body tag is great fun in the pool. The Judge (a great job for a parent) stands outside the pool calling out body parts, and the person who is It swims around trying to tag players on the chosen part.

CHAIN TAG (OR AMOEBA TAG)

In this version, when a player is tagged he or she must join hands with the person who is It. Play continues in this way until all players have been tagged by any player in the chain and have become part of the chain. The last player tagged becomes It for the next round.

CLOTHESPIN TAG

You'll want to raid the laundry room and stock up on clothespins for this novel variation. The clothespins are distributed evenly among all players (two to four per player is ideal). When the game starts, all players simultaneously try to "pin" each other. If each player was given two clothespins at the beginning of the game, being pinned twice leads to disqualification. The last player who remains unpinned is declared the winner. Of course, you'll want to remind players that pinning must be confined to clothing—not fingers, ears, or other body parts!

Playing for points. Instead of disqualifying pinned players, set a time limit for each round of play, allot more clothespins, and use a point system to determine the winner. Each time a player pins someone, he or she gets a point. The player with the most points at the end of the round is the winner. (Start with four clothespins each and make sure there's a spot where players who need them can get more.)

ELBOW TAG

You'll need an even number of players for this version of tag. All but two players spread around the field in pairs, with their arms hooked. One of the unpaired players is designated It, and the other is the first player to be chased. The player being chased can hook onto one of the pairs scattered on the field, in which case the second person in that pair becomes the chased. When someone gets tagged, the roles simply reverse. No immediate tag-backs are allowed.

FLOUR TAG

Gather some dark colored shirts, a few pairs of your mom's old pantyhose or stockings, and some flour to play this unique version of tag. Designate a "prison" area on the playing field using a garden hose or rope, and make sure it's large enough for all players to stand in at the same time.

Each player gets a pantyhose leg filled with about two cups of flour. The stocking should be tied off so the flour is in a compact ball at the end. Players tag each other by throwing these flour-filled stockings. Tagged players must go stand in the prison area, and the player who manages to stay flour-free is the winner.

Cleaning up between games. Tagged players will have a visible flour-mark on their shirts where they were hit, so it's important to clean up between rounds. Make sure to dust yourself off well, and use a damp cloth too, if necessary.

SHADOW TAG

This variation must be played on a sunny day. It chases the other players and tags them by stepping on their shadows. The player whose shadow was stepped on then becomes It. You can also designate safety bases (a tree, a fence) or "safety positions," such as dropping on all fours or touching your right shoulder to the ground.

A few hints. Players should stay as far apart as possible, to keep their shadows from overlapping. Also, remember that shadows are longer at sunset and toward evening than they are at midday.

TURTLE TAG

This variation is played just like basic tag, except there are no designated bases. To be safe from getting tagged, a player must lie on his back like an upside down turtle—but he can stay in that position only for a count of 10. This variation is especially well suited for very young children.

Be tricky. When you're It, chase one opponent and then quickly change direction to catch another player off guard. This sneak attack gives the players less time to fall down into the safe position.

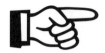

Blob Tag

Tag is easy enough to understand, and this version can accommodate players as young as kindergarten age. The neat thing is, the slower kids get to be part of the blob that chases the faster folks together, so it's almost fun to get caught first.

WHAT YOU NEED

* Any flat yard, park, or beach area that is a safe distance from traffic

HOW TO PLAY

* Choose one person to be the referee, and one person to be It.
* The referee should designate the boundaries, starting with about a half-acre (about half the size of a football field) and subtracting about 10 percent of the tag area as each new person is tagged.
* The person who is It counts to 10 and then starts trying to tag others. As each person is tagged, he or she must join hands with the person who is it, forming a "Blob."
* Each time the Blob gets bigger, the referee makes the field smaller, until only one person is being chased by the Blob, which is now made up of the rest of the players.
* When that last person is finally tagged, he or she becomes It to start the next round.

NO EQUIPMENT NEEDED

INDOOR OR OUTDOOR:
Outdoor

AGES:
5 and older

HOW MANY CAN PLAY?
At least 6, up to 10

WEATHER:
Warm and dry

TIME REQUIRED:
At least 20 minutes

PARENTAL SUPERVISION/ INVOLVEMENT:
Requires a referee-type

INTENSITY LEVEL:
Easy to moderate

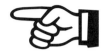

Band-Aid Tag

Beyond sheer physical exertion, tag can involve plenty of make-believe and role-playing. This game is fun and kind of like playing Twister on the run. Remember, as bad as it is to get tagged out, it's worse to get so tangled up you fall down...

WHAT YOU NEED

No equipment needed

SETTING UP

Choose a place far from traffic with at least 30 square yards of running space, such as the local park or a backyard with no slope. A few hilly spots and a few hard sidewalks are okay, but make them the exception, not the rule.

HOW TO PLAY

* Choose one person to be "Mr. Yuck." The other players run away (but they do not hide).
* If Mr. Yuck tags you, you have been wounded. You must cover the spot where he made contact (your "wound") with one of your hands as you continue the game.
* Should you get tagged a second time, you may cover your wound with your other hand.
* The third time you get tagged, you are out.

NO EQUIPMENT NEEDED

PERFECT FOR PARTIES

INDOOR OR OUTDOOR:
Outdoor

AGES:
5 and older

HOW MANY CAN PLAY?
3 or more

WEATHER:
Dry and above freezing; good warm-up game

TIME REQUIRED:
At least 15 minutes

PARENTAL SUPERVISION/ INVOLVEMENT:
Not necessary

INTENSITY LEVEL:
Moderate to Intense

TIPS FOR MR. YUCK

Try to tag people in places that will make it hard for them to run and cover the wound at the same time, such as the backs of their knees or the top of their head, or even their foot. Avoid the hips, waist, or upper thighs—covering a wound there will barely break someone's stride.

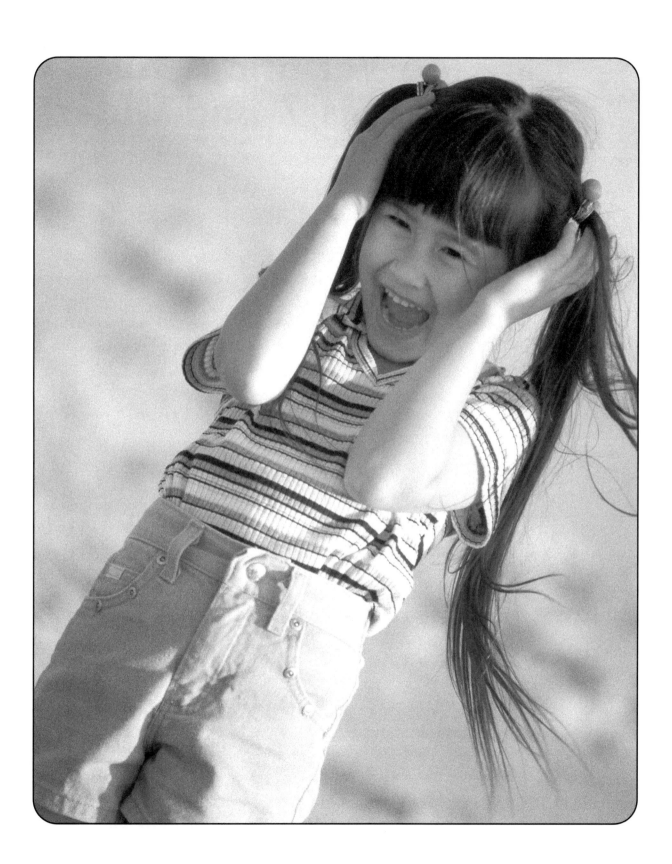

Tag Variations for Kids Ages 7 and Older

BLINDFOLD TAG

Because this variation is a bit more difficult, you'll want to designate a smaller playing area. The person who is It is blindfolded and runs around the playing field calling the names of other players. When a player hears his or her name, she has to answer, "Here I am!" The person who is It then tries to determine where the other players are based on how loud or soft their voices are.

Be sneaky. Try to get as close as possible to the person who is It without getting caught.

BROOM TAG

You will need a broom and at least four players for this version of tag. The player designated It is called the Broom Chaser and tries to tag other players with the end of the broom. Once tagged, the players become part of the Broom Chaser's team and have to help him capture the remaining players by grabbing on to them and yelling "Broom Chaser!" The Broom Chaser then comes and tags the player being held. The last remaining untagged player becomes the Broom Chaser during the next round.

FLASHLIGHT TAG

For this nighttime version of tag, you will need a flashlight. Once you have designated the safety base and chosen someone to be It, the remaining players scatter while the person who is It closes his or her eyes and counts to a 100 by fives. Players hide and try to sneak back to the safety base. If the person who is It shines the flash-light on a player, that player becomes It.

Blend into the night. Wear dark-colored clothing so that you are less visible in the dark.

Freeze Tag

In this spin-off, players must stop moving completely (freeze) when tagged. Players must remain immobile until another player "unfreezes" them, by either tagging them or crawling between their legs. Because the designation of It does not pass from one player to another during the course of the game, you should set a time limit of 10 minutes to 15 minutes. At the end of this period choose another player to be It.

Tunnel variation. Frozen types stay standing and can be unfrozen only if the unfreezing player crawls between their legs. (This works well for the under the age of 6 crowd.)

TV Tag

There are no safety bases in this version. Instead, the person who is It chases players who try to avoid being tagged. To keep from getting tagged, a player must kneel on the ground while saying the name of a television show—no repeats.

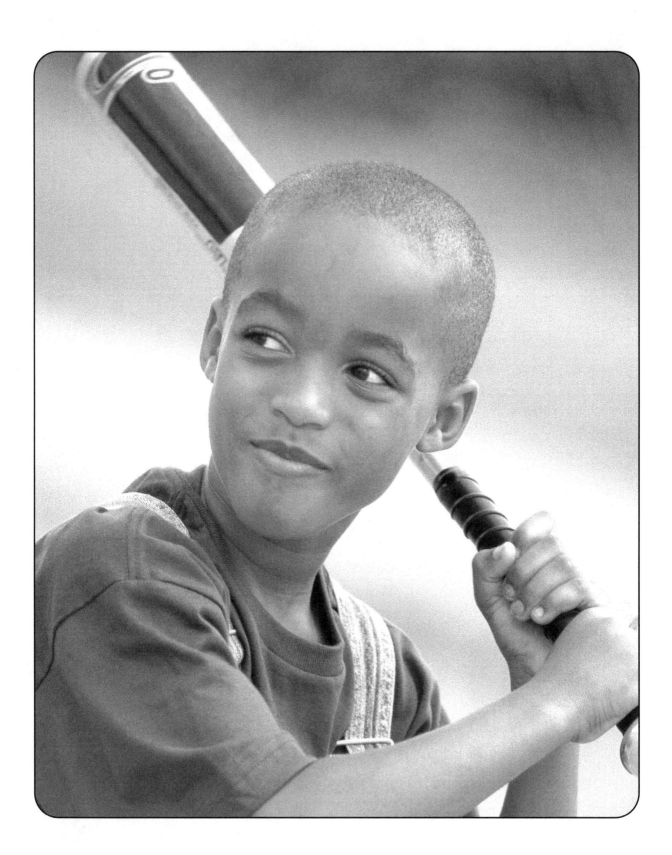

5

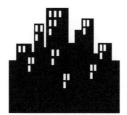

OUTDOOR GAMES IN THE CITY

TAKE THE FUN TO THE STREETS—AND THE SIDEWALKS

Grown-up city kids from L.A. to the Bronx have reminiscences all their own: Stickball, pitching pennies, Box Ball. Games invented on city streets require moxie and not much else. Most are played with a wall, some chalk, a ball, and maybe a stick. Though it's harder to come by a silent city street these days, you can still head for the sidewalk, the park, a vacant basketball court, or an apartment building courtyard to pass along these simple but engaging games to a new generation of city kids. And if you've never played them yourself, have you got a treat in store!

A GOLD MINE OF URBAN GAMES

The folks at streetplay.com have a "fantasy that thousands of people from the Boomer generation who grew up in urban America will love the stuff" in their site, which includes rules for all sorts of games from stickball and handball to skully—also known as bottlecaps. We have adapted a few of the classic games they celebrate on the streetplay.com website to fit the format of this book, including Hit the Stick and Stickball, and wish to acknowledge both their knowledge of the rules and their heartfelt attitude that all parents should share this street legacy with their kids. We strongly encourage you to visit streetplay.com for more games along with updates on tournaments and festivals (who knew Stickball had tournaments?) and fine reminiscences about the times "when it was okay to go outside, hang out with friends, and have a great time playing activities that didn't require a coach, schedule, or major amount of brand name equipment." Thanks, Streetplay!

Jump Rope

Jump rope is not just the all-time girl playground bonding game; it's aerobic exercise, once you catch on! And it improves coordination and grace, too. Don't present it as a feminine option, though, 'cause it's just as good for boys.

What You Need

❋ Jump rope 8 feet to 12 feet long

Setting Up

❋ Two players stand opposite each other on grass or on a sidewalk and swing the rope.

How to Play

❋ Two players swing the rope slowly until someone has jumped-in. They then gradually swing it faster while keeping a steady beat.

❋ Once someone has started jumping, the other players sing a rhyme while counting the number of successful skips made by the jumper(s).

Rules of Play

❋ The jumper's turn ends when she makes a mistake, or when the rhyme ends.

PERFECT FOR PARTIES

INDOOR OR OUTDOOR:
Outdoor

AGES:
5 and older

HOW MANY CAN PLAY?
3 or more

WEATHER:
Warm and dry

TIME REQUIRED:
At least 20 minutes

PARENTAL SUPERVISION/ INVOLVEMENT:
Not necessary, but it's nice if mom or dad will take a turn jumping or turning the rope

INTENSITY LEVEL:
Moderate to Active

✳ The winner is the player with the highest number of successful skips, or the largest number of completed rhymes.

JUMP ROPE RHYMES

Keep the beat with some of these fun jump rope rhymes.

Candy, candy in the dish. How many pieces do you wish? One, two, three, four, and so on (count until jumper misses).

Brent and Becky, sitting in a tree, K-I-S-S-I-N-G! First comes love, then comes marriage, then comes Becky with a baby carriage. How many babies did she have? One, two, three, four, and so on (count until jumper misses).

Cinderella, dressed in yella, went outside to kiss her fella. By mistake, she kissed a snake, came back in with a belly-ache. How many doctors did it take? One, two, three, four, and so on (count until jumper misses).

My little sister, dressed in pink, washed all the dishes in the kitchen sink. How many dishes did she break? One, two, three, four, and so on (count until jumper misses).

I went down town, to see Miss Brown. She gave me a nickel, to buy a pickle. The pickle was sour so she gave me a flower. The flower was black so she gave me a smack. The smack was hard so she gave me a card. And on the card it said:
Little dancer turn around (turn while jumping)
Little dancer, touch the ground (touch ground)
Little dancer tie your shoe (jump on one leg, pretend to tie shoe)
Little dancer, 64 skidoo (jump/exit rope area)

A player already jumping says, "I like coffee, I like tea, I like (another player's name) to jump with me." The person who was named jumps in. Then, the other players begin counting, "One, two, three, change places, seven, eight, nine, change places, and so on." Every time they group says "change places" the two jumpers must switch places without stopping. The other players keep track of who got the highest number of turns before missing.

MAKE A BOLA

It can get sort of boring to wait for a spin at the jump rope—and kids aren't being active while they're sitting around. If you don't have several jump ropes, try using a Bola. Before you can play you need to spend a little time making your own Bola. It's really easy—all you need is an old long tube sock, a rubber handball, a tennis ball (or another ball roughly that size), and a piece of rope (you can use a jump rope). Put the rubber ball into the sock, tie a knot right above the ball, and then tie your rope to the open end of the sock.

To play Bola, one player lies on the ground, grasps the Bola by the rope end, and starts spinning the Bola, slowly letting out the rope. When the spinner has the Bola rotating in a full circle, everyone can begin entering the circle to jump. The player on the ground can spin the Bola at varying speeds and heights to make the jumps more challenging for the other players. Anyone who gets hit by the rope is disqualified, and the game continues until only one player is left jumping.

Hit the Stick

Does all that video game-playing really improve your child's hand-eye coordination? Use this game as a test. You don't have to be fast or nimble to play Hit the Stick, but you do need good aim and some finesse.

WHAT YOU NEED

✳ Bouncy rubber ball such as a Spaleen (the lightweight balls sold in drugstores, toy stores, and urban delis)

✳ Eighteen-inch-long dry stick, stripped of branches. It shouldn't be too straight.

✳ Two adjacent sidewalk squares (like a ping-pong table pattern) or a similar pattern drawn with chalk on a driveway, courtyard, or basketball court.

SETTING UP

✳ Set the stick across the middle seam between the two sidewalk squares. Imagine setting up a ping-pong table, and place the stick where the net would go.

HOW TO PLAY

✳ Players stand behind the line of their sidewalk square, parallel to and facing the stick.

✳ Players take turns throwing the ball at the stick.

✳ Each hit scores one point. A player earns two points each time the stick flips over.

Rules of Play

❊ A player's feet must be behind the line when he or she throws, but bending is permissible.

❊ Play to 11 or 21 points, whatever you agree on ahead of time.

❊ If the ball moves the stick, the stick stays where it is for the next throw.

Soft-touch strategy. If the stick jumps closer to you, simply bend over and gently drop the ball to score a point. Once the stick is closer to you, keep throwing softly to give the other player a longer, more difficult shot.

A SWEET TRADITION

City kids will tell you that whenever possible, play for ice cream from the corner vendor—the loser buys for the winner.

HIT THE COIN

For this Hit the Stick variation, place a penny or nickel in the center seam instead of the stick, and check to see if it shows heads or tails. A player gets one point for hitting the coin and two points for flipping it over.

Hopscotch

Kids have been playing Hopscotch since the 1800s. That's not surprising, because Hopscotch is fun and easy to play and it doesn't require complicated or expensive equipment.

Hopscotch is a moderately physical game (although it can be modified to be more strenuous) designed for family members of all ages—unless you have trouble with balance, bending, or seeing well. It can be played outdoors in almost any weather, on sidewalks or driveways. When the weather doesn't cooperate, move a modified version of the game indoors, with a preprinted foam pad available for the purpose at most toy stores, if you like.

Hopscotch involves hopping, jumping, bending, stretching and balancing, providing a moderate aerobic workout while you take time to play together.

WHAT YOU NEED

* Chalk (for outdoor games)
* Masking tape or masking tape (for indoor games)
* Markers for each player (anything light that can be easily tossed; nothing round or breakable): large buttons, spoons, beanbags, small stones
* Hopscotch diagram
* Ten feet to 15 feet of flat ground

HOURS OF FUN

INDOOR OR OUTDOOR:
Both

AGES:
5 and older

HOW MANY CAN PLAY?
4 is the optimal number

WEATHER:
If outdoors, weather should be dry

TIME REQUIRED:
At least 30 minutes

PARENTAL SUPERVISION/ INVOLVEMENT:
Not necessary, but loads of fun

INTENSITY LEVEL:
Moderate. To increase the intensity of the game, quicken the pace, make the pattern larger, or play longer.

SETTING UP

✳ Once you've decided on a variation of Hopscotch you want to play (or have created your own) draw the diagram in chalk (for outdoor play) or in masking tape (indoor play), making each square 18 inches to 24 inches in size.

✳ Mark a starting line 6 inches to 12 inches from the first square of the Hopscotch diagram. The starting line can be drawn closer or farther away from the diagram to adjust the level of difficulty of the game. For example, it will be harder to toss the marker into box 8 if the starting line is drawn more than 6 inches from the Hopscotch diagram.

✳ In the most common version of hopscotch, the diagram is comprised of eight squares. Number the squares from 1 to 8 beginning with the square closest to the starting line.

✳ When deciding how large to make the diagram squares, consider the size and age of the children playing and each player's skill level. For example, if you're constructing a diagram for four first graders who are physically small but energetic, you would want to make the squares small enough so that the game is doable but large enough so that it's also challenging. On the other hand, if the group of children playing is more laid-back and less competitive, you would want to make the squares relatively small. This would allow for low-energy play that is still physical and fun, though less demanding.

✳ Creating a dome-shaped rest area on the far side of the Hopscotch diagram is optional and makes the game less physically demanding.

HOW TO PLAY

✳ After all players have chosen markers, Player 1 stands at the starting line and tosses his marker into square 1.

* Player 1 then hops over square 1 (where the marker is) onto square 2 and then continues hopping until he reaches square 8.
* At square 8, Player 1 turns around and hops back through the squares toward the starting line. When he reaches square 2 Player 1 bends down, picks up the marker from square 1, and jumps over square 1 out of the Hopscotch diagram.
* If Player 1 returns to the starting line without breaking any of the rules (see below) then his turn continues: From the starting line, Player 1 tosses his marker into square 2. He then hops into square 1, over square 2, and then through the rest of the squares as in the step above. Play continues in this manner until a rule is broken. It is then the next player's turn.

RULES OF PLAY

* A player must jump over the square with his marker in it. If the player fails to do this, his turn is over.
* All hopping must be done on one foot. The only time two feet can touch the ground at the same time is when the player reaches two side-by-side boxes in the diagram. In this case, the player must land with one foot in each square.
* A player is out if he fails to toss his marker in the appropriate square; for example, if he aims for square 3 but the marker lands in square 4.
* A player is out if he hops onto any line of the Hopscotch diagram.
* A player is out if he loses his balance when bending over to pick up a marker. Putting a second hand or foot down on the ground while bending is considered losing balance.
* A player is out if he lands in a single square with both feet.
* When a player is out he places his marker into the square where playing will resume on the next turn.
* The winner is the first player to advance his marker from square 1 to square 8, and then again from square 8 to square 1.

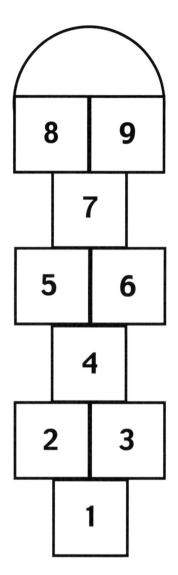

DRAW YOUR OWN PATTERN!

Use chalk to draw a hopscotch pattern on the ground, or use masking tape on a floor. The diagram should have 9 numbered sections. A dome-shaped "rest area" can be added on one end of the hopscotch pattern for the player can rest for a second or two before hopping back through.

Garage Volleyball

Simplicity itself: All you need for this game is a suburban garage or a city brick wall, a ball, a few interested folks, and a few minutes. Just remember to close the door first if you're one of the rare people who actually parks the car in the garage.

WHAT YOU NEED
* Fun Gripper Volleyball or rubbery playground ball
* Garage door, wall, or slanted roof

SETTING UP
You can play one-on-one or break into teams of two or three. Stand next to your teammates (if any) in a line across from the closed garage door or a hard, flat, clear exterior garage wall.

HOW TO PLAY
* One person, or a member of one team, bounces the ball against the wall volleyball style, with a closed fist or flat palm.
* Some member of the other team must then hit the ball back to the wall without catching or dropping it before it bounces on the ground.
* The volley continues, each team responsible for alternating hits, until someone lets it drop to the ground.

RULES OF PLAY
* If the serving team (or individual) drops the ball, that team loses the serve.
* If the other team drops the ball, the serving team receives 1 point.
* Play continues until one team reaches at least 15 points. The winning team must win by 2 points.

FUN FOR THE WHOLE FAMILY

HOURS OF FUN

INDOOR OR OUTDOOR:
Outside, next to the garage wall

AGES:
7 and older, or older depending on skill

HOW MANY CAN PLAY?
2, 4, or 6

WEATHER:
Cool or warm and dry (or nearly dry) concrete or asphalt driveway

TIME REQUIRED:
About 15 minutes per round

PARENTAL SUPERVISION/ INVOLVEMENT:
Not necessary

INTENSITY LEVEL:
Easy to moderate

Box Ball

This game is sort of similar to Four Square, but with a smaller, bouncy ball. This is a great game for two people waiting for the rest of a crowd—or for a parent and child who have a bit of extra time together.

What You Need

❋ A smallish rubber ball such as a Spaldeen (or, in a pinch, a tennis ball)

❋ Two connecting boxes (You can use concrete sidewalk boxes or draw sidewalk size boxes on an asphalt playground or driveway with chalk.)

How to Play

❋ Each person takes command of one of the two boxes. Players face each other across the line between the two boxes. They can stand either in the boxes or behind them.

❋ Hit the ball with your open hand, directly into the opposite box.

Rules of Play

❋ You score a point if your opponent can not return the ball within one bounce and keep it inside your box.

❋ Whoever loses the point starts the next volley.

HOURS OF FUN

INDOOR OR OUTDOOR:
Outdoor

AGES:
7 and older

HOW MANY CAN PLAY?
2 players or 2 players per side

WEATHER:
Cool or warm and dry (or nearly dry) concrete or asphalt court

TIME REQUIRED:
15 to 30 minutes per game

PARENTAL SUPERVISION/ INVOLVEMENT:
Not necessary

INTENSITY LEVEL:
Moderate

Slow-Pitch Stickball

Baseball lore says that Willie Mays was a fearsome Stickball player. He was known as a "four-sewer man," meaning he could hit the ball four sewer manholes away from home plate (a stickball home run if ever there was one). While Stickball enthusiasts may debate the truth of that story, they all agree that Stickball is a fast and fun game. If you played when you were a street urchin, get out there and show the kids how it's done. If not, pick it up alongside them.

What You Need

✳ A bouncing rubber ball such as a Spaldeen (the ideal)
✳ A stick (the straight end of a broken ice hockey stick or a broom stick is best)
✳ A quiet street or asphalt playground or paved schoolyard

Setting Up

Create a baseball style field with a home plate, three bases, and a "foul" zone.

How to Play

✳ Typical baseball rules apply. Batters hit the ball and then run the bases.

* The pitcher stands about 30 feet away from the hitter and delivers a sidearm lob (with some spin) that the hitter tries to clobber on a single bounce.

RULES OF PLAY

* If a batter takes three swings without a fair hit, he or she is out.
* If a pitcher throws four balls outside the strike zone, the batter gets an automatic walk to first base.
* Certain violations result in automatic outs. Stickball purists insist that anything that lands on a roof must be an automatic out. Of course, anything that breaks a window or lands on a porch or area that gets players in trouble is also an automatic out. (Although breaking a window might qualify as an "automatic side-retired.")

SAMPLE STICKBALL DESIGNATIONS

A group that bills itself as the Amateur Stickball League doesn't actually run bases for slow-pitch or Fungo Stickball (See page 138), instead preferring to use these designations:

Single. Any ball hit on the ground past the pitcher, but fielded by an outfielder. Also, any fly ball that takes a bounce before it is in the outfielder's hands. If a player is hit with a pitch he or she is awarded a free trip to first. Four balls pitched outside the strike zone and not hit by the batter are equal to a single.

Double. Any fly ball that hits an outfielder (anywhere on his or her body) without being caught is a double. Any ball dropped by an outfielder attempting to catch the ball, or any ball on a fly that goes over the head of the outfielder and hits the ground without hitting the back fence, is a double. If the ball hits the pitcher and then hits the ground, it is a double.

Triple. Any ball that hits any spot on the back wall or fence on the fly is a triple. If the ball is fielded by the fielder directly off the wall or fence, it is not an out.

Home Run. Any ball that goes over the back fence is a home run, even if the ball hits the top of the fence before it goes over. If a player goes around the fence and catches the ball, it is considered a home run. The person who hits a home run is responsible for the ball and must go and get it.

Foul Balls. Any ball hit on or to the right of the "baseline," whether that's a sidewalk or a line in the dirt, is considered a foul. Any ball that bounces in front if the pitcher's mound (assuming the pitcher has not touched it) is a foul ball. Any player who hits a foul ball has to find it and bring it back to the game.

Double Play. If there is a base runner on first and batter grounds out or flies out to the pitcher, it is considered a double play. If playing wall ball, the pitcher also has to throw the ball against the strike zone (the blue box on the wall). If the pitcher elects not to throw the ball at the strike zone or misses the strike zone, the runner is considered safe at first.

Stickball Diagram

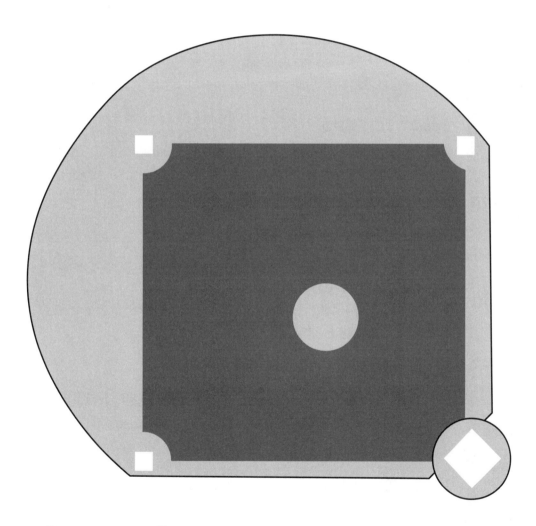

BATTING IN THE DIAMOND

A stickball field resembles the typical baseball diamond. Four "plates" are set evenly spaced apart, surrounding the pitcher in the center of the field, creating as close to a ninety-foot square as possible.

Fast-Pitch Stickball

● ●

**FUN FOR THE
WHOLE FAMILY**

PERFECT FOR PARTIES

BIG GROUP FUN

HOURS OF FUN

INDOOR OR OUTDOOR:
Outdoor

AGES:
7 and older

HOW MANY CAN PLAY?
3 or more

WEATHER:
2 teams, ideally 3 to 4
per team

TIME REQUIRED:
30 minutes to 2 hours,
depending on the
number of innings

**PARENTAL SUPERVISION/
INVOLVEMENT:**
Yes, until you're sure
the area is safe

INTENSITY LEVEL:
Moderate to intense

This version is also known as Wall Ball—and as the name implies, it requires you to pitch the ball against the wall.

WHAT YOU NEED

❋ A bouncing rubber ball such as a Spaldeen (the ideal)
❋ A stick (the straight end of a broken ice hockey stick or a broom stick is best)
❋ A quiet street or asphalt playground or paved schoolyard
❋ A wall that can serve as a backstop. If you have chosen a parking lot, make sure there are no cars parked between the playing area and the wall.
❋ A concrete field of play that is at least 10 yards long and the width of a driveway.

SETTING UP

❋ Draw a "strike zone" on the wall with chalk. It will be the same for all players (instead of the baseball tradition, between a player's armpits and his or her knees across the width of home plate), so try to give the shorter kids a break by making it reasonably sized. A good start might be from the waist to the shoulders of the shortest player, across the width of home plate.
❋ Choose landmarks or mark distances that determine whether a hit is a foul, single, double, triple, or homer. (See typical layout for Stickball, page 135.) Batters

won't actually run the bases, you'll just keep track of their progress and scoring.

HOW TO PLAY

❋ Divide into two teams of up to three players. The team that will play in the "outfield" first should determine who will pitch and who will field (no base defenders are required.)

❋ The pitcher stands a few yards away from the batter and throws an overhand pitch to the batter, who stands in front of the wall.

❋ If the batter hits the ball and no one catches it on the fly, the batter earns bases depending on the distance the ball travels.

RULES OF PLAY

❋ The pitch must not bounce before it reaches the batter.

❋ If a batter swings and misses at two pitches, he or she is out.

❋ If a pitcher throws three pitches that fail to bounce off the strike zone on the wall, the batter gets a "walk" to first base.

❋ Fouls count as strikes.

❋ No grounders allowed.

❋ Once a team has three outs, the other team is up.

TIPS FOR PITCHERS

The way to get better at Wall Ball is to practice when no one is around. Just keep throwing the ball against the wall, trying to put it in the strike zone.

Fungo Stickball

Fungo is now the most common style currently played among organized Stickball leagues. (Yes, there are organized Stickball leagues!) Fungo follows the same rules as slow-pitch for the most part. The twist is that you pitch to yourself.

What You Need
* A bouncing rubber ball such as a Spaldeen (the ideal)
* A stick (the straight end of a broken ice hockey stick or a broom stick is best)
* A quiet street or asphalt playground or paved schoolyard

Setting Up
* Create a baseball style field with a home plate, three bases, and a "foul" zone.

How to Play
* Typical baseball rules apply. Batters hit the ball and then run the bases.

Rules of Play
* If a batter takes three swings without a fair hit, he or she is out.
* It's legal to let the ball bounce more than once before hitting it.

HOW TO SELF-PITCH:

Here's a quick lesson in the fine art of self-pitching.

1. Toss the ball in the air with one hand and hold the stick with other.
2. Let the ball bounce once as you grab the stick with your other hand, too, and prepare to slug the ball.
3. As the ball rises into your strike zone, swing the stick to smack it out of the park.

Of course, it is legal to let the ball bounce two or three times before you swing, but it won't bounce as high and you are not allowed to retoss it.

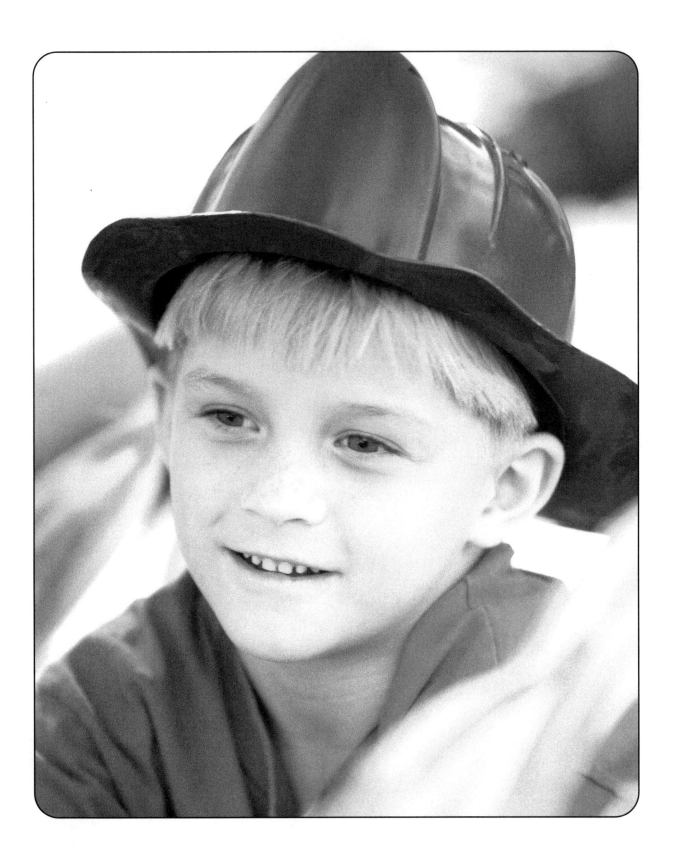

6

OUTDOOR GAMES IN THE SNOW

Fun When It's Freezing

OUTDOOR GAMES THAT CURE CABIN FEVER

Don't let snowfall and subfreezing temperatures keep you inside. Just adapt ordinary games to chilly conditions, and you can have fun all year round. Here are some snow games at every activity level to get you started.

Snow Hurdles

Track and field events may seem like strictly summer fare, but it's fun to run and jump in the snow, too. Enlist the kids in sculpting the hurdles for this snowy course, and they'll get two bouts of exercise—and two chances for fun. Just make sure you set up the course only in soft, not ice-covered, snow, because hurdlers are bound to take some spills.

WHAT YOU NEED

✳ Potting soil
✳ Shovel for snow

SETTING UP

✳ In a snow-covered yard, vacant lot, neighborhood park or schoolyard, form snow walls at least 4 inches thick, 2 feet wide and 1 foot tall. These are your "hurdles," so be sure to space them along a trail of unbroken snow that the children can run across easily, and space them at least 5 feet apart so that the runners can easily land from one jump before having to work up momentum for the next.

✳ Use a couple handfuls of potting soil to mark a start and finish line 5 feet from the first and last hurdles.

✳ Possible trail shapes include a straight line, oval or circle, figure eight, heart, snowman shape, or one child's first initial.

HOW TO PLAY

✳ Draw names for starting order, and let runners take turns running the course alone. Run for fun or try one of the following competitive variations.

FUN FOR THE WHOLE FAMILY

PERFECT FOR PARTIES

BIG GROUP FUN

HOURS OF FUN

INDOOR OR OUTDOOR:
Outdoors

AGES:
Can be adapted to any age older than 3

HOW MANY CAN PLAY?
The whole neighborhood

WEATHER:
At least 3 inches of snow on the ground, but not icy

TIME REQUIRED:
At least 30 minutes; set up is part of the activity

PARENTAL SUPERVISION/ INVOLVEMENT:
Need 1 older person to set up

INTENSITY LEVEL:
Moderately active

Snow Hurdle Variations

REVERSE LIMBO
Each time all the hurdlers have successfully cleared the hurdle course, add a couple inches of snow to the top of each hurdle. Runners are eliminated if they can't clear all the hurdles without touching the tops. The one who completes the course with the highest hurdles wins.

TWO LANES
For this version, you must create two snow hurdle courses side-by-side. Two players race each other to successfully complete the course—without touching or knocking over the hurdles.

TAKE YOUR TIME
If the snow—and the hurdles—will be around for a few days, so can this game. Using an inexpensive stopwatch or the second hand on your wristwatch, time kids running through the course—and keep a running record in a notebook or on a memo pad. If you like, give little trinkets for each time a child improves his time by 3 seconds. This is a nice chance to help kids understand the concepts of improving their personal best and competing with themselves instead of others. This variation even works with relay teams. Keep track of a team's personal best by running relays and giving rewards (or gold stars!) when the whole relay manages to cut its time by 5 seconds or more.

BUILD AND GO
In the hours after a big snowstorm, especially when the plow hasn't made it through yet, round up the gang for a course-building relay. Divide into two teams and give each team leader the desired dimensions of the course (say, five hurdles spaced 5 yards apart). Who wins? The team that builds and runs the course successfully first.

Ice Cube Hunt

INDOOR OR OUTDOOR:
Outdoors

AGES:
Three and up

HOW MANY CAN PLAY?
2 to 10

WEATHER:
Very cold, but not if the weatherman is issuing cautions about the cold

TIME REQUIRED:
At least 30 minutes, plus time for the ice cubes to freeze

PARENTAL SUPERVISION/ INVOLVEMENT:
Need 1 older person to set up

INTENSITY LEVEL:
Easy to moderately active

Why wait for Easter? Make an afternoon of searching for colorful, small objects—and then go have hot chocolate, instead of chocolate bunnies. This hunt is perfect for all ages, and will bring the most jaded outside for at least a few minutes. If you have a few kids who feel they're "too old" for such shenanigans, enlist them to hide the cubes, because that will get them moving, too.

WHAT YOU NEED

* ❄ Food coloring
* ❄ Ice cube trays
* ❄ Lots of hiding spaces
* ❄ Plastic bowls

SETTING UP

* ❄ Make batches of different colors of water (at least red, yellow, blue, and green, but you can also experiment) and then use them to freeze at least five trays of ice cubes.
* ❄ While the "hunters" stay inside where they can't see what's going on, a willing adult or teen hides the ice cubes. (Note: If you have a mixed age group, make sure to put some near the ground, some at each person's eye level, and some where only the bigger kids will see them.)

How to Play

✳ Give each hunter a plastic bowl in which to collect cubes.

✳ Call everyone together to explain which parts of the yard contain cubes, and which are off limits.

✳ After everyone is bundled up, release the hunters one at a time, youngest to oldest, allowing 10 seconds lead time between hunters.

✳ The person to find the most colored ice cubes is the winner.

PURPLE CUBE EXTRA

For fun, make just one purple cube and tie a particular award to it. If you are playing with family, you might say that the person who finds the purple cube can skip a night of doing the dishes, for example. If the players are a group of friends, you can offer a monetary award, such as one dollar.

Snow Tag

A favorite with the Boy Scouts, this is a gleeful game of hot pursuit. If you make a big wheel pattern in the snow, the players will run a lot. If you make the wheel smaller, the action will be faster and more players will get a chance to be It. Consider making two circles so that you can play either way. Purists know to play in deep snow, because it's impossible to go out of bounds with the snow heaped there, and you can't run or even walk very quickly with snow banks surrounding you.

What You Need

❄ Shovel for snow

Setting Up

❄ In a fairly flat yard or vacant lot of unbroken snow, tramp out a circle at least 15 feet in diameter. The circle can be larger if you want more exercise and the people playing are pretty fast runners. Make the path around the perimeter at least 8 inches wide, but not wider than 1 foot or it's too easy to run.

❄ Without making any other footprints, walk off a straight path across the circle. Then make two more intersecting paths across the circle to cut it into six equal pie wedges. (From above, it should look like a bicycle wheel with six spokes.) Again, make sure not to disturb the snow between the paths.

HOW TO PLAY

❋ The person who is It takes his place at the center of the wheel.

❋ The other players scatter around the rim of the circle (not on the spokes).

❋ The person who is It asks, "Ready?" When the other players all confirm with, "Ready!" the game begins.

❋ The person who is it sets off, darting down one of the spoke paths to try to tag another player.

❋ If the person who is It tags someone, he or she must hold on to that player long enough to repeat, "Snow Wag, Snow Rag, Snow Tag!" Then the tagged person becomes It, and heads to the hub of the wheel to start the game again.

RULES OF PLAY

❋ Two players cannot pass each other on the narrow paths.

❋ If you cut it too close and fall into the snow off the paths, you're fair game to be tagged.

❋ If a player leaves the path, he immediately becomes It.

❋ If the person who is It leaves the path, he or she loses the chance to play in that round and must stand outside the playing area. The other players choose a new person to be It.

Ice Age Tug-of-War

Try this Tug-of-War variation to stretch those winter-weary arm and leg muscles—and to laugh and roll around with friends. Be sure to warm up and do some stretches first, and make the teams as even as you can—balancing number, weight, and strength of players—if you want the game to last longer.

What You Need

✳ A snowy patch of earth that's at least 20 feet by 20 feet
✳ Two old polyester-blend sheets

Setting Up

✳ Tamp down a shallow trench across the middle of your snowy patch. The trench should be about 2 inches deep, 2 feet wide, and 6 feet long.
✳ Tie knots in the sheets, lengthwise, at 2-foot intervals.
✳ Tie one end of one sheet to one end of the other to make an 8-foot to 10-foot "rope" you can grasp with gloved hands.

How to Play

✳ Divide the players into two teams and designate a leader for each.

* The leaders of each team should face each other across the mid-point of the trench (but not standing in the trench), with their teammates lined up single file behind them.
* Each team gets to hold precisely half of the sheet "rope"— with the center extending across the trench.
* At the "Go!" signal, both teams grasp the "rope" and pull, in an attempt to tug the other team's members into the trench.
* Whichever team pulls the other team entirely through the trench and on to their team's side (along with the rope, naturally) wins.

RULES OF PLAY

* The sheet rope can't touch the ground.
* All players on the team must be grasping the rope at all times.

Sledding Snow Target

If you are lucky enough to get a lot of sledding weather, keep it interesting by setting up this snowy shooting range—shooting snowballs, that is. This is for people who are used to sledding and can control a sled easily, so not just anyone can play, and a parent or responsible adult should monitor the game closely at first for safety reasons. You'll want to make sure the kids aren't losing control of their sleds or crashing into each other. Plus, if you're right there, you'll get a workout too, because who can resist throwing snowballs on the move?

WHAT YOU NEED:
* Buckets
* Sledding hill
* Sleds
* Snow
* Snowballs

SETTING UP
* Set buckets, right side up, along a course down the sledding hill. Be sure to choose a course that your players can sled without too much difficulty. Put the buckets at least 5 feet away from each other, so the player has a chance to pick up another snowball before passing too many buckets.

HOW TO PLAY

✳ Give each player two snowballs at the top of the hill.

✳ As each sleds down the hill, he or she should try to toss the snowballs into the buckets.

✳ A player gets one point for hitting the bucket and two points for successfully tossing the snowball into the bucket.

RULES OF PLAY

✳ No stopping on the way down.

✳ If you fall off your sled, that turn is over and you take your place at the top of the hill.

✳ The game's lowest-scoring contestant must take the highest-scoring contestant's sled up the hill for him three times after the game is over.

OTHER TARGET IDEAS

No buckets in the house? Use any of the following as targets.

Bushel baskets

Plastic basketballs pressed 1 inch into the snow (three points if you can hit it hard enough to roll down the hill)

Plastic shoe-storage size organizing boxes with lids

Plastic waste-paper baskets, bathroom size

Small snowmen (score extra point for hitting the snowman on the head)

Three pieces of firewood set in a triangle

Twins

What kid hasn't wanted to be a "twin" with a best friend or a near lookalike at some point in his or her young life? Play on that, and play hard, with this sprinting game. If some players are getting all the action, break into two circles or make a rule about taking turns.

WHAT YOU NEED

❄ A park, large back yard, or other large area.

HOW TO PLAY

❄ Pair off all players into sets of "twins," then join hands to form a large circle.
❄ One set of twins is chosen to be the runners.
❄ The runners jog around the outside of the circle and tag a pair of joined hands. Then the runners run in one direction around the circle, as quickly the tagged twins break out of the circle and run around it in the opposite direction.
❄ The first pair back to the vacated spot gets to keep the spot, and the other pair becomes the new runners.

TIP FOR SAFE PLAY

Make sure to set up rules for passing so that no one gets hurt. For example, make the runners always pass on the outside or the "twins" have to duck so the others can jump over them.

NO EQUIPMENT NEEDED

INDOOR OR OUTDOOR:
Outdoor

AGES:
8 and older

HOW MANY CAN PLAY?
6 or more

WEATHER:
Warm and dry, or snowy

TIME REQUIRED:
At least 20 minutes

PARENTAL SUPERVISION/ INVOLVEMENT:
Not necessary

INTENSITY LEVEL:
Moderately active to intense

Crack the Whip

This game is a great option for active kids, and involves a bit of strategy too, to avoid getting "cracked" by the force of the "whip." The true risk-takers can try it on ice (remember the scene with Snoopy in *A Charlie Brown Christmas*?), but the rest should stick to firm, not hard, earth.

WHAT YOU NEED

No equipment needed.

SETTING UP

* Players line up in a large backyard covered in several feet of fresh, powdery snow and hold hands tightly.
* The player on one end of the line is the "head," while the player on the opposite side is the "tail."

HOW TO PLAY

* The player at the head of the line starts running quickly—twisting and turning at will and pulling the rest of the players along with him.
* When the player reaches top speed he "cracks the whip" by stopping suddenly, making the players at the tail of the line go flying.

NO EQUIPMENT NEEDED

PERFECT FOR PARTIES

INDOOR OR OUTDOOR:
Outdoor

AGES:
9 and older

HOW MANY CAN PLAY?
6 or more

WEATHER:
Snowy, or warm and dry

TIME REQUIRED:
At least 20 minutes

PARENTAL SUPERVISION/ INVOLVEMENT:
Not necessary

INTENSITY LEVEL:
Moderately active to intense

RULES OF PLAY

✳ Play safely. The force generated by cracking the whip can be very strong, so players at the tail should be prepared for the abrupt stops.

✳ The person at the head of the line should be a relatively strong player.

TIPS FOR SAFE WHIP-CRACKING

When your gang is playing Crack the Whip, keep these tips in mind.

✳ The player at the tail should hold on tightly with both hands, and still be prepared to go flying.

✳ Check that there are no dangerous objects (rakes, lawn furniture) on the playing field and that there is plenty of open space for the whip to crack.

FUN IN THE SUN
Try this game in the summer, in a large, grassy backyard.

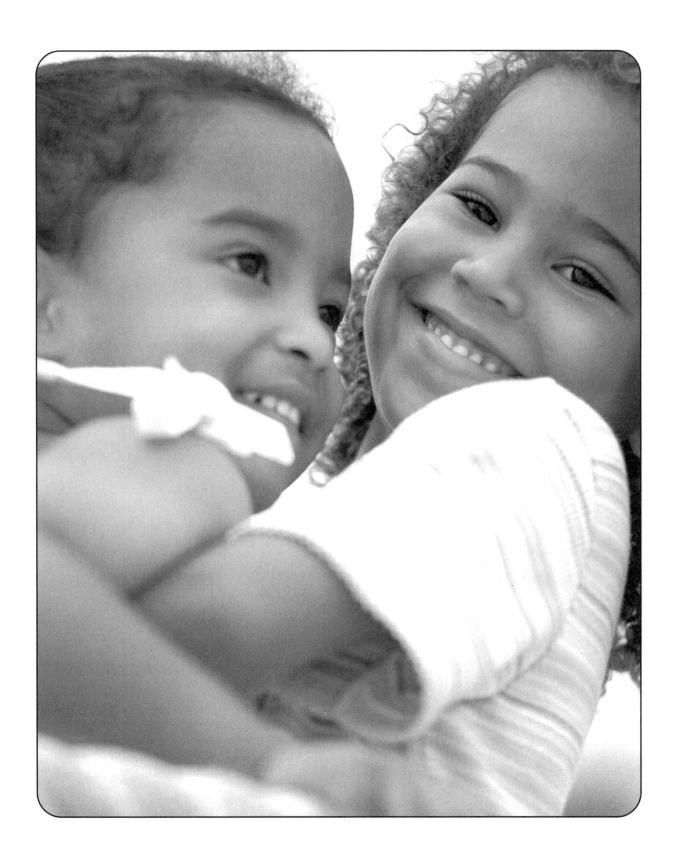

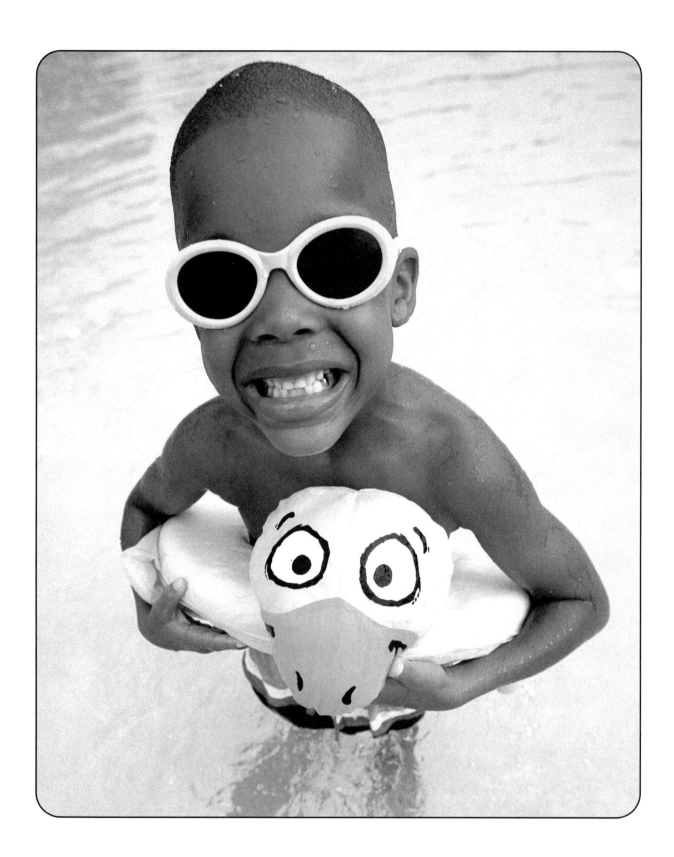

1

OUTDOOR GAMES IN THE WATER

Whether you're already outside for the day and looking for entertainment or want to lure folks from the TV in the sweltering months, think H2O. Nothing brings out the glee like soaking your mom—or your wife—with a water balloon! These games will help you organize the chaos a bit, and give your picnic in the park or day at the pool something fun to focus on. Just remember basic water safety rules, including no diving in shallow water, running on wet grass, or holding people underwater. Then, get drenched and be happy!

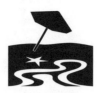

Frozy Toesies

Even in this day of home saunas and Olympic-size health club pools, the humble wading pool can draw crowds in the first steamy days of the season. Add another simple pleasure to the mix with this simple game, fun for preschoolers and a hoot for adult parties too.

What You Need

* Wading pool
* Several trays of ice cubes with plastic jacks frozen inside

Setting Up

* The day before you want to play, freeze several trays of ice cubes with one plastic jack (or other small plastic toy or ring) inside.
* Fill the wading pool with cool water.
* Just seconds before play starts, dump the ice cubes in the water.

How to Play

* Each player tries to get as many ice cubes as she can out of the pool—using just her toes and feet!

Rules of Play

* If you pick up an ice cube with anything but your toes or feet, you must return it to the pool and forfeit two more too.
* If any of the players is substantially younger or smaller than the others, he gets to start a full minute before the others (or adjust according to age difference and ability).

SUPER-QUICK

PERFECT FOR PARTIES

INDOOR OR OUTDOOR:
Outdoor

AGES:
3 and older

HOW MANY CAN PLAY?
3 or 4

WEATHER:
Warm if you're near a hot shower, otherwise very hot

TIME REQUIRED:
About 10 minutes

PARENTAL SUPERVISION/ INVOLVEMENT:
At least for the first round

INTENSITY LEVEL:
Moderately active

Bucket Brigade

A nice cooperative game that might prepare your child for future work as a volunteer fire fighter... or as a slapstick comic. Lots of running, so consider water shoes if the grass gets slick. A great game to play if it's high time you watered the lawn.

What You Need

* Plastic wading pool and an outdoor source of water
* Grassy back yard or field at a park
* Two large buckets like the ones paint or birdseed come in
* One smaller bucket for each player, including plastic beach pails, large to-go cups, sour cream tubs, etc.

Setting Up

* Set the wading pool at one end of the yard and fill it with water.
* Mark a "full" line inside each of the larger buckets, about 5 inches from the top, then set them down about 20 yards from the wading pool and about 10 feet apart.
* Divide into two teams.
* Have each team line up single file, with the first person standing next to the wading pool and the last next to the team's large, empty bucket—and all the players holding their individual buckets.

BIG GROUP FUN

INDOOR OR OUTDOOR:
Outdoor

AGES:
4 and older

HOW MANY CAN PLAY?
4 to 12

WEATHER:
Warm to hot

TIME REQUIRED:
At least 20 minutes

PARENTAL SUPERVISION/ INVOLVEMENT:
Helpful, but a responsible preteen can handle it

INTENSITY LEVEL:
Moderately to fairly active

How to Play

* At a predetermined signal, the two players closest to the pool fill their buckets and pour the water into the next player on their team's bucket.
* The water continues down the line, brigade-style, and the final player in the line pours it into the larger bucket.
* The first team to fill the bucket wins.

Rules of Play

* Before any water can be poured into the large bucket, it must be poured into and out of each member of the team's bucket.
* No one is allowed to pick up the empty bucket.
* Players have to hold their individual buckets in their hands and stand up—no sitting or placing the buckets on the ground.

Strategies for Success

* If you have different-size individual buckets, make sure the youngest (or the least competent) players get the ones with the largest openings.
* Put your strongest players nearest the wading pool so you don't lose a lot of water right at the start.

Variations

* If you're playing with a mixed-age crowd, require adults to "walk" on their knees.
* To prolong the game, make a rule that only one pail of water can make the rounds at a time.
* To make the game more active, have the person who pours the water into the empty bucket then sprint back to the wading pool and join the front end of the line.

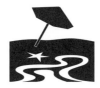

Marco Polo

Every time a gang gathers at a neighborhood or indoor pool, scare up a game of Marco Polo. The object is not to be tagged by the unseeing It, and lots of splashing, scurrying, and fake voices are part of the fun. Make sure to adhere to all water safety rules, though. One person should just watch the game, and no running on deck, dunking, or dive bombing (particularly the one with her eyes shut). This is also a game where it's good to be little and quick, a perfect time to put little kids and athletic adults on equal footing.

What You Need

✳ Indoor pool
✳ Light blindfold

Setting Up

✳ One person is chosen to be It and he or she dons the blindfold or closes their eyes and moves to one end of the swimming pool.

How to Play

✳ It ducks under water and counts to 10 and bursts up to the surface and shouts, "Marco."
✳ All the others in the pool shout, "Polo" and it tries to figure out where they are in the pool based on their response.

INDOOR OR OUTDOOR:
Outdoor

AGES:
5 and older

HOW MANY CAN PLAY?
4 or more

WEATHER:
Warm to hot
(or indoor pool)

TIME REQUIRED:
At least 15 minutes

**PARENTAL SUPERVISION/
INVOLVEMENT:**
Yes

INTENSITY LEVEL:
Easy

* It can repeat the shouting as many times as he likes, all the while trying to tag one of the other players.
* If a player gets tagged, she becomes It and play continues.

RULES OF PLAY

* It can never remove the blindfold or open his eyes.
* Players cannot restrict each other's movements, or touch or jump in on It. If someone does, they're out entirely for two rounds.

FAST TRAVEL VARIATION

To make the game more active, add a rule that anyone except It can sneak out of the pool, though they still have to answer if It calls, "Marco" and only one person can do this at a time. When It suspects that someone's out of the water, she shouts "Spaghetti" and the one caught out becomes It. If it's a false alarm, It has to play with one hand behind his back for the next minute.

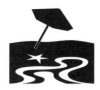

Trash Target

Kind of a mix between the dunking booth at the school fair and a no-blades Medieval battle, this game uses mostly stuff you have around the house. It's great for just two or an energetic crowd, and it reinforces agility and hand-eye coordination. If your kid needs prep for playing goalie or isn't real confident at dodge ball, this game is great training.

WHAT YOU NEED

❊ Fifty to 100 water balloons
❊ Rain gear or large trash bags, bathing suits or water-ready clothing
❊ Two extra large trash can lids
❊ Chalk or string to form a box for "target" players to stand in

SETTING UP

❊ Prepare the water balloons and stash them in a bucket or laundry basket.
❊ Mark two 5-foot diameter circles about 5 yards apart.
❊ Divide into two teams.
❊ Line up facing the other team, with the first person in each line outfitted in rain gear and holding the trash can lid like a shield, standing inside the box.

HOW TO PLAY

✳ Flip to see which team will throw first.

✳ The first player on the team that wins the draw gets three water balloons. She stands in the circle drawn for her team and tries to hit the first player in the facing circle with successive water balloons, waiting for the first balloon to hit or miss the player before launching another.

✳ The player on the other team tries to defend himself by wielding the trash can lid. If the balloon hits the target player on the body, the thrower's team gets one point. If the balloon is deflected, the target's team gets a point.

✳ After three balloons, the players switch roles and scoring continues.

✳ When the first pair's turn is over, they step off to the sidelines or to the back of the line and play continues with the next pair.

RULES OF PLAY

✳ If a "target" player steps out of the circle, his team loses a point.

✳ Players must go in order and no player can have a second turn until all players have taken their first turn.

✳ Play to 25 or whatever score you agree on ahead of time (or as many balloons as you have).

Hoppin' H$_2$O

Here's a great option for those scorching summer side-walks—set up a game of water jump rope. You can play any place there's a hard surface and two people willing to turn the rope. Best of all, the novelty of the water might be enough to lure your kid into learning how to jump rope, which is a fantastic form of aerobic exercise and also builds confidence and coordination.

WHAT YOU NEED

* Long playground-style jump rope
* Two small paper cups for each contestant
* Garden hose or 2-liter bottles of water
* Clothes that can get wet or bathing suits
* Old tennis shoes or water shoes (no flip flops or bare feet for safety's sake)

SETTING UP

* Decide who will turn the jump rope—they should be good and consistent so each child has a fair turn.
* Fill the water glasses.
* Choose the jumping order.

HOW TO PLAY

* One at a time, the contestants attempt three jumps in a row holding the two cups of water.
* Whoever has the most water left in their cups when everyone's had their turn wins. Or, you can keep play-ing until only one contestant has water left in a cup.

FUN FOR THE WHOLE FAMILY

INDOOR OR OUTDOOR:
Outdoor

AGES:
6 and older, or younger if a kid can jump rope

HOW MANY CAN PLAY?
2 to 6

WEATHER:
Warm to hot

TIME REQUIRED:
At least 20 minutes

PARENTAL SUPERVISION/ INVOLVEMENT:
Need two competent turners

INTENSITY LEVEL:
Moderately active

Close Shave Shootout

Screeching fun for elementary school kids, this messy water fest might also draw teens and rowdy adults. You'll need a little skill, a lot of water guns, and at least one player on each team who's not faint of heart. Ready, aim... fun!

WHAT YOU NEED

* Can of shaving cream
* Outdoor source of water
* One water gun per team
* Clothes that can get wet or bathing suits

SETTING UP

* Determine how many teams you want—each must have a water gun and a member who's willing to get wet and doesn't mind if water gets on her face. Divide into teams.
* Choose the person from each team who will serve as target and spray a circle of shaving cream on the front of her shirt, making sure each team has the same amount and size.
* Have the target members form a row 5 feet from their teammates. Draw or set a "foul" line 5 feet from each "target" player for the "shooters" to stand behind.

BIG GROUP

FUN FOR THE WHOLE FAMILY

PERFECT FOR PARTIES

INDOOR OR OUTDOOR:
Outdoor

AGES:
6 and older

HOW MANY CAN PLAY?
6 to 20

WEATHER:
Warm if you're near a hot shower, otherwise very hot

TIME REQUIRED:
At least 20 minutes

PARENTAL SUPERVISION/ INVOLVEMENT:
At least for the first round

INTENSITY LEVEL:
Moderately active

How to Play

✱ Players from each team take turns standing behind their team's foul line and using the water gun to try to shoot the shaving cream off their "target" teammate's shirt.

✱ The team that succeeds first wins, although other teams get a final turn to try to even the score if they haven't had as many shots as the successful team.

Rules of Play

✱ If a shooter crosses the foul line, her team loses their next shot.

✱ If water from one team's gun hits another team's target player, they forfeit their next turn.

✱ All players on each team must shoot in turn and no one can be skipped.

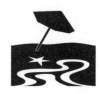

Wet T-Shirt Relay

FUN FOR THE WHOLE FAMILY

PERFECT FOR PARTIES

SUPER-QUICK

INDOOR OR OUTDOOR:
Outdoor

AGES:
6 and older

HOW MANY CAN PLAY?
6 or more at least
10 preferred

WEATHER:
Warm and sunny

TIME REQUIRED:
At least 15 minutes

PARENTAL SUPERVISION/ INVOLVEMENT:
Yes

INTENSITY LEVEL:
Active

This isn't what you think! You play with bathing suits on! It's lots of fun and lots of finagling, perfect for a pool party or summertime family reunion.

What You Need

＊ One bucket of water per group
＊ One XXL T-shirt per group
＊ Bathing suits
＊ Water shoes or old shoes for all (bare feet are okay on the sand)

Setting Up

＊ Draw a starting and finish line about 20 yards apart, placing a base or post at the end of each.
＊ Divide into two teams and form lines about 3 yards apart with a full water bucket at the starting line.
＊ Give the dry T-shirt to the first person on each team.

How to Play

＊ At the agreed on "go" signal, the first person on each relay dunks the T-shirt into the bucket of water, puts it on, runs down to tag the base and runs back to give the T-shirt to the next person in line, who must be standing behind the starting line.
＊ The next person repeats the drill and so on until all on the relay have run. The first group to finish wins.

Rules of Play

✳ Each player must put the T-shirt over his head and his arms through both sleeves before he can start running.

✳ Any player who doesn't touch the base before returning to the starting line must retrace her route and touch the base.

✳ Any player who takes off the T-shirt before passing the finish line must go back to the base and put it on again before proceeding.

✳ If the teams are uneven, the other team may choose who runs twice to even the score.

✳ All decisions of the judge are final.

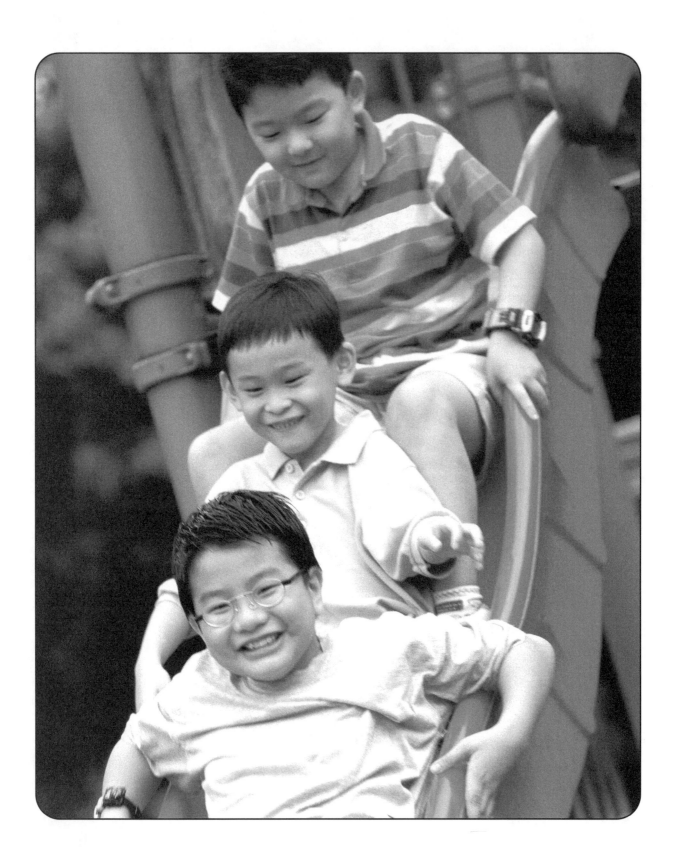

CONCLUSION

. . . .

"The years pass by too quickly it seems," says the old Peter, Paul and Mary song, and I would have to agree. Just in the time since I began collecting these fitness games for publication, my trio of little girls have become teenagers, more intent on eye makeup than sidewalk chalk these days, more interested in walking the mall than playing Follow the Leader.

Sometimes I get sentimental thinking that they may never spend hours in the hot sun entertained only with a plastic bat and ball, three flip flops acting as bases and their benevolent stepbrother serving up easy pitches. But I remind myself that they're still active, Kristen with soccer and Y basketball, Lucy with swing dance and climbing, Frances with karate and occasionally riding and mucking stalls at a local horse stable.

And just as I get too teary about spent childhoods, there is my super-serious 13-year-old climbing trees with her Science Olympiad friends waiting for the carpool, or my high schooler demands that everyone get up from the video games and go play Capture the Flag at an annual Halloween party.

My kids aren't wealthy, but I think they're the lucky ones. Whether it's good genes or all that Duck, Duck Goose played at day care, they're reaping the critical benefits of an active lifestyle. Not only does activity decrease body fat and increase muscle mass, it lowers blood pressure and reduces stress, which combats the depression that seems to loom as a possibility for any teen. It's reassuring to me that for my kids moving and playing are already an ingrained habit, one that will probably help them cope.

One of our favorite joking topics is my daughter's elementary school gym coach. After days of drills and jogging, she told the class they were going to get to play a game! My daughter, primed by life at our house, was wild with anticipation. But the game was . . . Fitness Kickball. The teams counted off and lined up like they would for ordinary kickball, only if you made a kick for your team, you got to choose which calisthentic everyone did while you ran the bases—pushups, jumping jacks, or situps.

How fortunate that my child knows how funny that is, how much more fun activity should be, can be. And any parent who will take the time can give their child this free luxury—a life filled with games and motion. You'll find that it gives you a boost, too, a chance to be a playmate for a change, some time to forget about grown-up stress for a few minutes.

Of course, there's no guarantee about fitness in later life. But with options like Amoeba Tag, water balloon toss, and Mother, May I? in the repertoire, what's the worst thing that can happen? Your family will make memories, that's what. And your kids will get to be kids for a time, and there's nothing better than that.

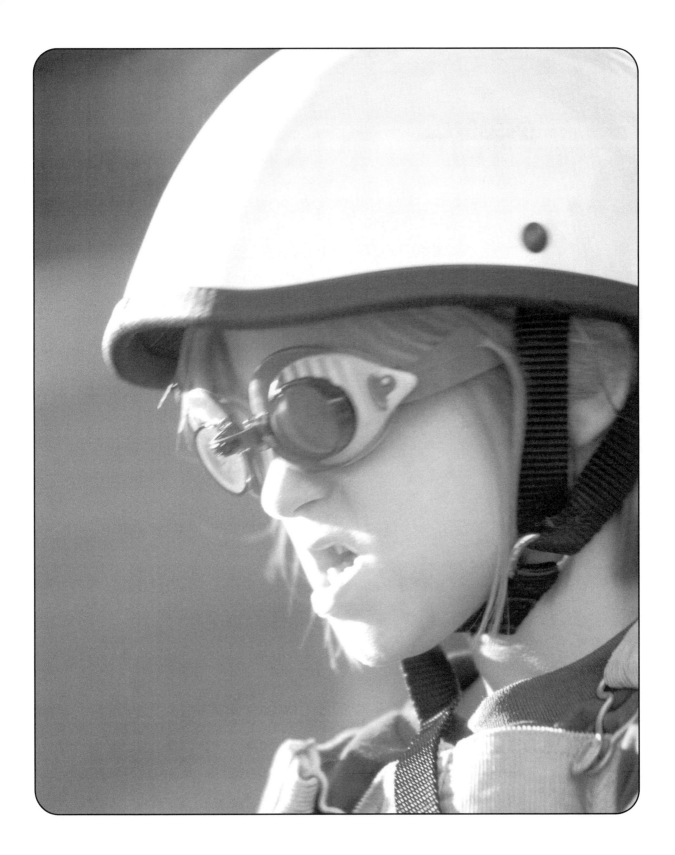

RESOURCES

If family fun equipment isn't readily available in your local discount department store, let your fingers do the walking (or the typing on your keyboard) to these Internet resources. At the end is a list of websites that deliver the latest data on youth fitness, which you can use to motivate your family to get moving—or to make the benefits of what you're already doing more tangible.

MANUFACTURERS

Spalding
spaldeen.com
Makers of Spaldeen balls.

Wham-O
wham-o.com
Makers of Frisbee flying saucers and other toys for indoor and outdoor play.

Hasbro
hasbro.com
Makers of Nerf balls and other toys for indoor and outdoor play.

ORGANIZATIONS

Outward Bound
www.outwardbound.org
A non-profit educational organization with programs in the wilderness, urban settings, workrooms, and classrooms.

President's Council on Physical Fitness and Sports
www.fitness.gov
An advisory committee of volunteer citizens who advise the President about physical activity, fitness, and sports in America.

Shape Up America
www.verbnow.com
The Center for Disease Control and Prevention's program to get kids more active.

INDEX

T

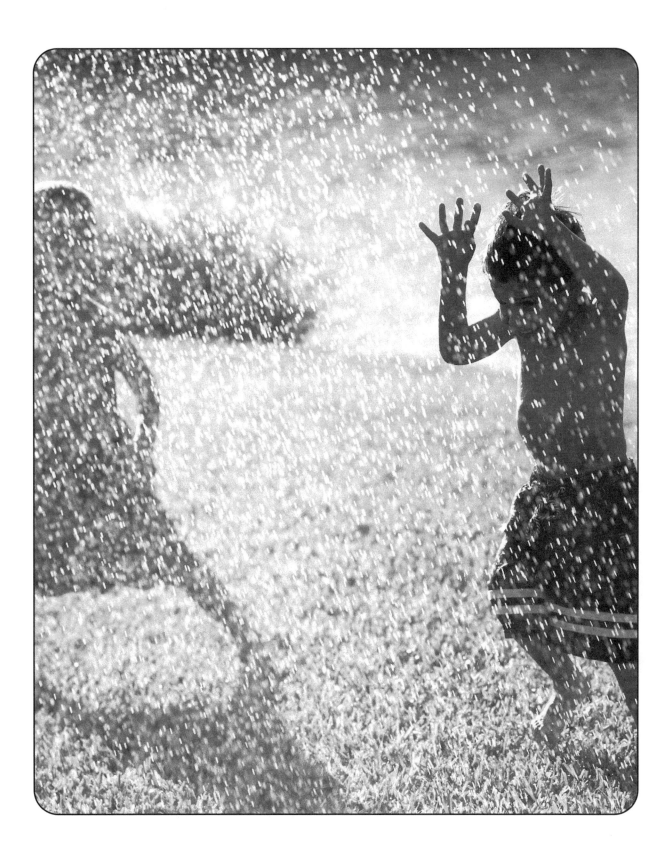

ABOUT THE AUTHOR

Rose R. Kennedy has a B.A. in English from the University of Virginia and regularly contributes to the cable television Fine Living Network's website and frugal living how-to books. A juvenile and kids' book reviewer since 1991, Rose annually interviews 10 best-selling authors for the Disney Adventure magazine kid-voted book awards.

The seventh of eight Baby Boomer siblings, Rose has 22 nieces and nephews, most of whom participated in her recently organized Family Reunion Olympics, with events ranging from an outdoor spelling bee to a hula hoop longevity contest. She has worked as a communications consultant and employee events planner. She has coached for the non-competitive American Youth Soccer Organization since 2000 and led three co-ed middle school soccer teams to winning seasons.

She lives in Knoxville, Tennessee with three still-active teenage girls who are known to play Capture the Flag on occasion.